An Atlas of Investigation and Diagnosis
OSTEOARTHRITIS

An Atlas of Investigation and Diagnosis

OSTEOARTHRITIS

Adrian Jones

Nottingham City Hospital
Nottingham, UK

Michael Doherty

University of Nottingham
Nottingham, UK

CLINICAL PUBLISHING

OXFORD

Distributed worldwide by
CRC Press
Boca Raton   London   New York   Washington D.C.

Clinical Publishing
An imprint of Atlas Medical Publishing Ltd
Oxford Centre for Innovation
Mill Street, Oxford OX2 0JX, UK

Tel: +44 1865 811116
Fax: +44 1865 251550
Web: www.clinicalpublishing.co.uk

Distributed by:

CRC Press LLC
2000 NW Corporate Blvd
Boca Raton, FL 33431, USA
E-mail: orders@crcpress.com

CRC Press UK
23–25 Blades Court
Deodar Road
London SW15 2NU, UK
E-mail: uk.tandf@thomsonpublishingservices.co.uk

© Atlas Medical Publishing Ltd 2005

First published 2005

All rights reserved. No part of this publication may be reproduced, stored in a retrieval system, or transmitted, in any form or by any means, without the prior permission in writing of Clinical Publishing or Atlas Medical Publishing Ltd.

Although every effort has been made to ensure that all owners of copyright material have been acknowledged in this publication, we would be glad to acknowledge in subsequent reprints or editions any omissions brought to our attention.

A catalogue record for this book is available from the British Library

ISBN 1 904392 16 4

The publisher makes no representation, express or implied, that the dosages in this book are correct. Readers must therefore always check the product information and clinical procedures with the most up-to-date published product information and data sheets provided by the manufacturers and the most recent codes of conduct and safety regulations. The authors and the publisher do not accept any liability for any errors in the text or for the misuse or misapplication of material in this work.

Printed in Spain by Fisa - Escudo de Oro SA, Barcelona

Contents

Abbreviations	vi
Preface	vii
Acknowledgements	vii
1 *Introduction*	1
2 *General features of osteoarthritis*	31
3 *Subsets of osteoarthritis*	41
4 *Features of osteoarthritis at specific sites*	53
5 *Principles of management*	95
Appendices	101
Index	103

Abbreviations

AADA apatite associated destructive arthritis

ACR American College of Rheumatology

ANKH ankylosis human (gene)

BCP basic calcium phosphate (crystals)

BMI body mass index

CMC carpometacarpal (joint)

CT computed tomography

COX cyclooxygenase

CPPD calcium pyrophosphate dihydrate (crystals)

DIP distal interphalangeal (joint)

DISH diffuse idiopathic skeletal hyperostosis

MCP metacarpophalangeal (joint)

MRI magnetic resonance imaging

NSAIDs non-steroidal anti-inflammatory drugs

OA osteoarthritis

PIP proximal interphalangeal (joint)

WOMAC Western Ontario and McMasters Universities (Index)

Preface

Osteoarthritis is the commonest joint disorder, being more prevalent than all other forms of arthritis added together. No book is fully comprehensive, but we hope that this *Atlas of Investigation and Diagnosis* will prove of interest to doctors and allied health professionals who manage people with osteoarthritis, and will act as a catalyst to encourage interest in this, the most common single cause of lower limb disability in the elderly.

Adrian Jones
Michael Doherty

Acknowledgements

We are very grateful to Jonathan Gregory for his support and perseverance in commissioning this book. We are also indebted to the Arthritis Research Campaign for infrastructure funding (Integrated Clinical Arthritis Centre [ICAC] grant), and for substantial funding of osteoarthritis research in Nottingham. Our academic co-ordinator, Helen Richardson (ICAC funded), as always played an essential role in organizing the authors.

Chapter 1

Introduction

What is osteoarthritis?

The answer to this apparently simple question is an ongoing problem for a condition that is so common. Everyone seems to be able to recognize 'osteoarthritis' when they see it, but, as with many rheumatological conditions, providing clear-cut diagnostic criteria has proved more difficult. Notwithstanding problems of definition, it is widely accepted that osteoarthritis is the most common condition to affect synovial joints, and is responsible for a great deal of pain and disability. Although a universally accepted definition has proved elusive, there is general agreement on some of the hallmark features of osteoarthritis. Cartilage loss is universally observed in all patients with osteoarthritis and, as will be discussed further below, is a *sine qua non* for diagnosis. Cartilage loss tends to be focal rather than widespread throughout the joint, particularly in the early stages of osteoarthritis (**1.1**).

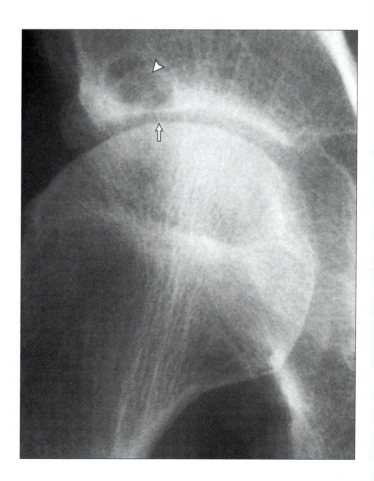

1.1 X-ray of a hip showing focal cartilage loss (joint space narrowing) (arrow) in the superior aspect of the joint. Note also the prominent acetabular cyst (arrowhead).

Bone response with increased bone formation adjacent to the joint is also commonly observed although, as discussed later, this varies in prominence at different joint sites and between patients (**1.2–1.4**).

Bone response may manifest itself as either as osteophytosis or subchondral bone sclerosis. These two features (i.e. cartilage loss and bone response) have often been considered the main features of osteoarthritis, but, as will be discussed later, it is now clear that many other tissues are involved in osteoarthritis. Indeed, it is likely that these other tissues are more important in determining the symptomatic and functional consequences of osteoarthritis. (*Table 1.1*, **1.5**).

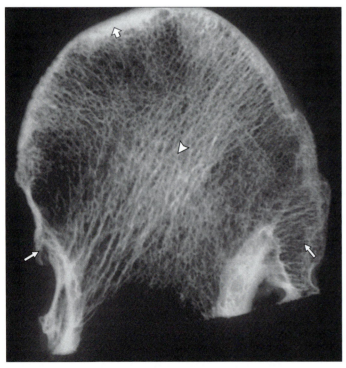

1.2 Slab radiograph of femoral head section from an osteoarthritic hip joint, showing marginal new bone (osteophyte) (arrows); thickening and increased whiteness (sclerosis) of the superficial subchondral bone (short arrow); and thickening of the trabecular arcades in response to altered stress loading (arrowhead).

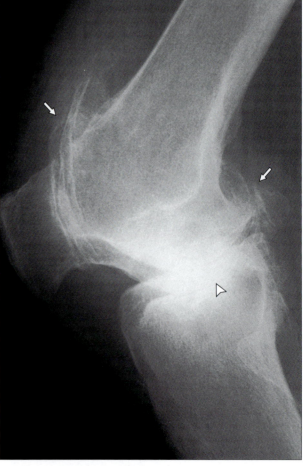

1.3 Hypertrophic patellofemoral osteoarthritis. Note florid new bone (osteophyte) formation at the joint margins (arrows) and sclerosis (increased bone density on x-ray) in the subchondral bone (arrowhead).

Introduction

Table 1.1 Tissues involved in osteoarthritis

Cartilage	Focal softening and loss
Bone	Osteophyte, sclerosis, but subchondral osteopenia
Capsule	Thickening
Synovium	Thickening and modest inflammation
Muscle	Atrophy and weakness
Ligaments	Degeneration
Bursae	Secondary bursitis
Vessels	Angiogenesis, avascular necrosis, venous hypertension

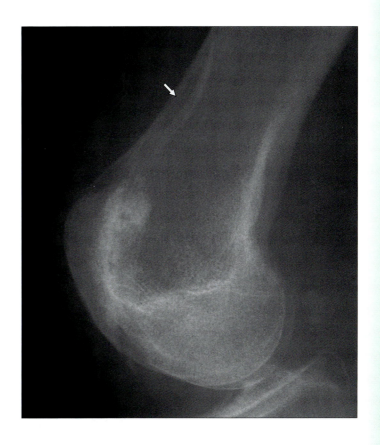

1.4 Atrophic patellofemoral osteoarthritis. Note loss of bone stock and relatively little osteophyte formation. Also note the apparent 'pressure erosion' (arrow) in the anterior aspect of the distal femur, as if the patella has scalloped out the bone and worn it away.

1.5 Diagram showing some of the major changes that occur in osteoarthritis.

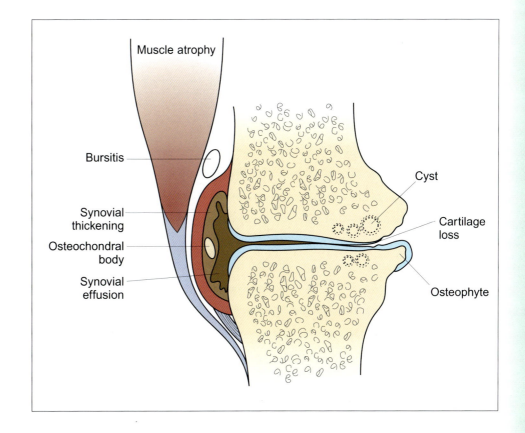

4 Introduction

The history of osteoarthritis

In order to understand the concept of any disease, it is necessary to look at its historical context. It is likely that osteoarthritis has been present throughout human history. Indeed, it may be of significant evolutionary importance, and this is discussed further below (page 29). The first attempts to describe 'arthritis' generally did not distinguish inflammatory from non-inflammatory disease (1.6). Gouty arthritis was probably the first specific arthropathy to be characterized, followed by infective arthritis and rheumatoid disease.

The reduction in infectious diseases as a result of public health measures, and the introduction of effective therapies for inflammatory arthritis, have resulted in an increased awareness and interest in non-fatal, but disabling diseases, such as osteoarthritis. In the 1950s, the introduction of the widespread use of radiography enabled ready study of diseases (such as osteoarthritis) which principally affect bony structures.

The combination of these factors resulted in an increased awareness of the impact of osteoarthritis, and enabled the conduct of large-scale epidemiological studies of this disease.

The next boost to the study of osteoarthritis came with the development of animal models of osteoarthritis and, in particular, the Pond–Nuki model of osteoarthritis – the anterior cruciate-deficient dog. The importance of this model is that it allowed study of the factors involved in the development of osteoarthritis. This, and other animal models, led to the realization that osteoarthritis is an active metabolic process, rather than a simple eburnation and erosion of cartilage. It also ultimately led to the realization that many other tissues, especially the neuromuscular system, are crucially important in the development of osteoarthritis.

Improved biochemical and cellular techniques further developed interest in the metabolic features of osteoarthritis, although arguably it may have led to an initial undue emphasis on cartilage.

In the 1980s and 1990s, a re-exploration of the epidemiology of osteoarthritis resulted in a renewed appreciation of the fact that not all patients with osteoarthritis are symptomatic. This is an obvious fact to anyone who looks at community samples of osteoarthritis, but can easily be overlooked in an outpatient setting where all patients have been referred because of symptoms. The implications of this has important consequences for understanding the epidemiology of osteoarthritis, and is discussed further below (page 29).

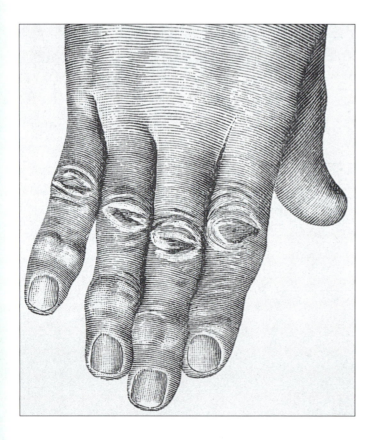

1.6 Nineteenth century drawing of a hand affected by nodal osteoarthritis prior to formal description of the condition (Charcot, Paris).

More recent developments in osteoarthritis have followed from the observations of the metabolic activity of osteoarthritis tissues and the realization that these processes may be amenable to modification by pharmaceutical means. This is more fully discussed in the section on disease modification (page 99). It has meant, however, that the pessimistic view that osteoarthritis is inevitably progressive has been challenged, and there is increasing pharmaceutical interest in manipulating this process.

The realization that osteoarthritis is the cause of significant health care expenditure, and that use of these resources may not always be rational, has led to increased health service research in this area, and the development of care pathways and guidelines for the management of osteoarthritis. The principles that have emerged from such endeavours are discussed in Chapter 5.

Finally, it is important not to forget that, in parallel with this, there has been immense interest in surgical interventions for osteoarthritis. These have included osteotomy, arthroplasty with increasingly complex prostheses, and, more recently, arthroscopic approaches, including tissue transplantation.

The epidemiology of osteoarthritis

The epidemiology of osteoarthritis has been elucidated by a number of major cross-sectional studies (pathological, clinical, and/or radiographic). There have also been a number of prospective studies of varying duration which have also illuminated our knowledge. Due to this, a number of risk factors and associations have been identified.

Other species

Osteoarthritis appears to have been present throughout our evolutionary history and, indeed, in many current non-human species. Looking across species, it is clear that all animals that fuse epiphyses of synovial joints are capable of developing osteoarthritis. The few often quoted exceptions (e.g. bats and sloths) probably simply reflect lack of study rather than any specific species difference (**1.7**). This has several important implications. Firstly, it allows potential study of mechanisms of osteoarthritis in non-human, non-primate species which can thus enhance understanding. Secondly, it probably implies that the biological processes that underlie osteoarthritis are most likely of great evolutionary value to the host organism. This has led some to speculate that osteoarthritis is an aspect of the inherent repair process of the joint, and has led to the coining of the term 'regenerative' joint disease.

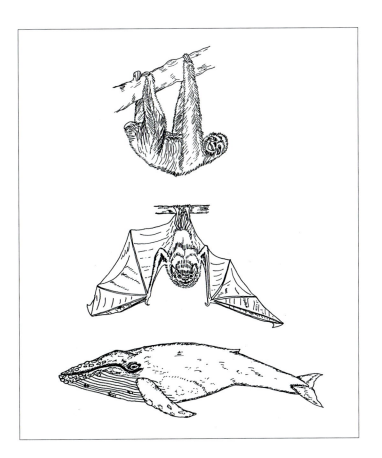

1.7 Although only minimally studied, osteoarthritis has been said not to occur in sloths and bats because they hang upside down and place distraction forces, rather than impact forces, through their joints. However, whales can develop osteoarthritis even though their weight is supported in water. It seems that osteoarthritis affects most species that have synovial joints and which fuse their epiphyses in the adult.

Age

All studies clearly define that the prevalence of osteoarthritis increases with age at nearly all joint sites (**1.8**). Obviously, since osteoarthritis, once established, demonstrates permanent changes in the joint, some of this could be regarded as the simple accrual of new joint involvement. However, there is a rapid rise in the prevalence of osteoarthritis after the age of 40. This occurs at all synovial joints, although the absolute prevalence varies at different joint sites.

Some forms of osteoarthritis are more likely to develop at specific ages. For example, osteoarthritis of the distal interphalangeal joint is uncommon before the age of 40, but polyarticular onset around the time of the menopause is common with a period of rapid accrual in the decade either side of 50 years of age.

There is a suggestion that the prevalence of osteoarthritis may even decline in the very elderly. These data derive from cross-sectional surveys and, of course, may reflect a survival effect (censureship) in that osteoarthritis may associate with premature cardiovascular mortality.

Gender

A number of studies have demonstrated that the relative prevalence of osteoarthritis at different joint sites differs between genders, usually being more prevalent in women. Both polyarticular osteoarthritis of the distal interphalangeal joints ('nodal generalized osteoarthritis') and knee osteoarthritis are more common in women than in men. At other joint sites, this sex difference is less dramatic and may differ with age. For example, hip osteoarthritis is more common in men before retirement age, but becomes more prevalent in women in older age.

Animal studies have confirmed that sex hormones can have a major effect on the development of osteoarthritis. Studies in humans have, however, only hinted at an effect on osteoarthritis, and a therapeutic use for sex hormones has not been demonstrated.

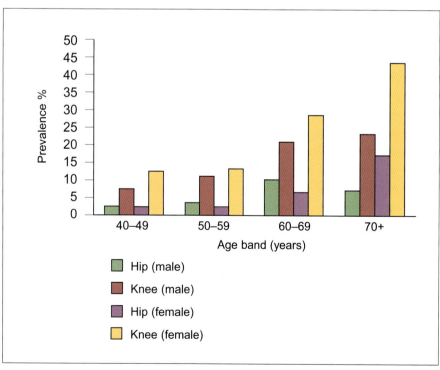

1.8 Prevalence of osteoarthritis at the hip and knee and in men and women by age. (Data derived from van Saase JL, van Romunde LK, Cats A, *et al.* [1989]. Epidemiology of osteoarthritis: Zoetermeer survey. comparison of radiological osteoarthritis in a Dutch population with that in 10 other populations. *Ann Rheum Dis,* **48**:271–280.)

Obesity

At most joint sites, but particularly the knee, weight has an important impact on the development and severity of osteoarthritis (**1.9**). More importantly reduction of weight in obese and overweight adults has been shown in a prospective observational study to reduce the subsequent development of knee osteoarthritis (**1.10**).

How obesity and overweight lead to the development of osteoarthritis is not entirely clear. The most likely explanation is mechanical overloading. The support for this comes from a study that has demonstrated that obesity interacts with malalignment at the knee (either varus or valgus) to increase the risk of developing radiographic osteoarthritis.

A counter to the simple mechanical argument is that obesity is acting through a metabolic mechanism. The main support for this proposal relates to hand osteoarthritis. It is argued that hand joints are 'non-weight bearing'. Therefore, the mechanism of the observed increase in hand osteoarthritis seen in the obese must relate to an associated metabolic imbalance. A number of possible mediating factors have been suggested including insulin-derived growth factor. However, it may not be that straightforward since mechanical studies have shown that forces through the hand joints in the obese are substantially increased.

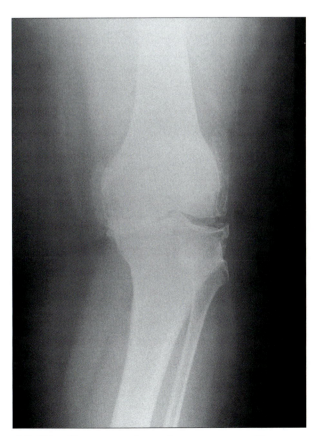

1.9 Standing x-ray of an obese woman with severe medial tibiofemoral osteoarthritis and varus malalignment. The soft-tissue shadows clearly illustrate this important risk factor for knee osteoarthritis.

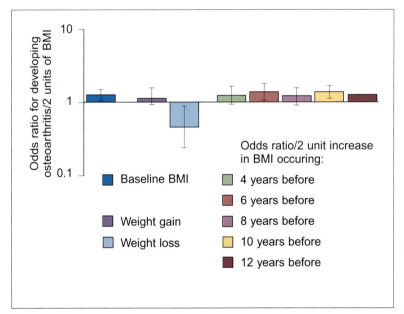

1.10 Effect of obesity on the subsequent development of knee osteoarthritis, and the additional effect of losing or gaining weight in the preceding 10 years. (Data derived from Felson DT, Zhang Y, Anthony JM, et al. [1992]. Weight loss reduces the risk for symptomatic knee osteoarthritis in women. The Framingham study. Arthritis Rheum, **116**:535–539.)

8 Introduction

Trauma

It has long been suspected that severe trauma to a synovial joint might predispose to subsequent osteoarthritis. Support for this comes from clinical observation of patients who have suffered fractures and who subsequently develop osteoarthritis of an adjacent joint (**1.11**). The risk of such 'secondary' osteoarthritis is particularly high when a fracture involves the articular surface of a joint.

Additional evidence comes from follow-up of patients who have undergone meniscectomy at the knee (**1.12**). Removal of a meniscus is a major mechanical insult to the knee and post-meniscectomy subjects are at increased risk of premature osteoarthritis on the side of the meniscectomy (**1.13**). The lifetime risk of developing osteoarthritis may not be increased, but the time of onset certainly does seem to be brought forward.

The degree of trauma required to increase the risk of subsequent osteoarthritis is unclear. However, a recent prospective study of college students suggests that even relatively minor trauma, insufficient to lead to hospitalization, is still associated with an increased risk of knee osteoarthritis in young adult life.

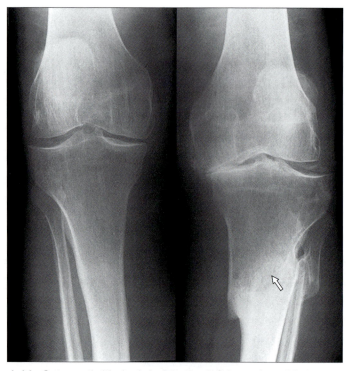

1.11 Osteoarthritis isolated to the left knee in a 64-year-old man who, 25 years before, had suffered a severe upper tibial fracture (arrow), resulting in leg length shortening and altered biomechanics. Note also bilateral chondrocalcinosis.

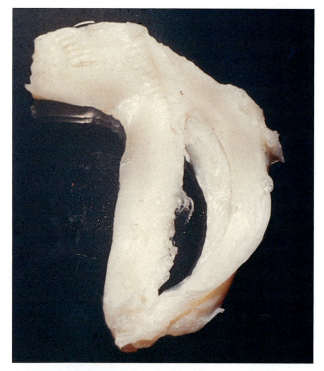

1.12 A longitudinal 'bucket-handle' tear of the medial knee meniscus. Tears of the medial meniscus are three times more common than lateral tears.

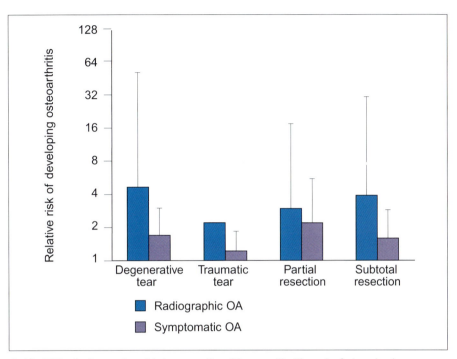

1.13 Effect of meniscal injury on the 16-year likelihood of developing osteoarthritis. (Data from a case-control study by Englund M, Roos EM, Lohmander LS [2003]. Impact of type of meniscal tear on radiographic and symptomatic knee osteoarthritis: a sixteen-year follow up of meniscectomy with matched controls. *Arthritis Rheum*, **48**:2178–2187.)

Genetic

An important genetic contribution to development of osteoarthritis has been suggested by classic twin and family studies. Strong heritability was first noticed for generalized nodal osteoarthritis, characterized by the presence of multiple Heberden's nodes. These nodes were described by William Heberden in 1802 in his *Commentary on the History and Cure of Disease*:

'What are those little hard knobs, about the size of a small pea, which are frequently seen upon the fingers, particularly a little below the top, near the joint? They have no connection with the gout, being found in persons who never had it; they continue for life; and being hardly ever attended with pain, or disposed to become sores, are rather unsightly, than inconvenient, though they must be some little hindrance to the free use of the fingers.' (Heberden W [1802]. *Commentarii de Morborum Historia et Curatione*, London.)

As will be discussed later, this form of osteoarthritis generally has its onset in perimenopausal women, hence its other common name of 'menopausal arthritis'. It shows strong inheritance, particularly in women, and behaves almost as a sex-linked, autosomal-dominant condition.

Other rare forms of atypical, young-onset osteoarthritis, often with minor degrees of dysplasia, have been described which transmit as monogenic disorders. In some families, the precise genetic association has been identified as mutations of the gene COL2A1 that encodes Type II collagen – the principal structural collagen of hyaline articular cartilage. However, investigation of patients with more common 'sporadic' osteoarthritis has failed to find such mutations as a common cause. Such reports in families have, however, fuelled interest in the genetics of more common forms of osteoarthritis.

More recent genetic epidemiology studies, using a variety of strategies (**1.14**), have confirmed an important genetic component to the development of osteoarthritis at a number of sites including the hip, knee, hand, and spine. The heritability of osteoarthritis at these sites (that is, the degree of variance for osteoarthritis in the population that is explained by genetic factors) is estimated to be between 40–60%. Linkage and association studies continue to try to identify the responsible genes (**1.15**). Although a number of findings are reported, most have not been replicated in subsequent studies. It is clear, however, that osteoarthritis is a common complex disorder, and that several, possibly even multiple genes, will contribute to susceptibility. These are likely to be common polymorphisms rather than mutations; they may vary according to joint site, and they may need to interact with other genes, or with other constitutional or environmental risk factors to express the phenotype of osteoarthritis (**1.16**).

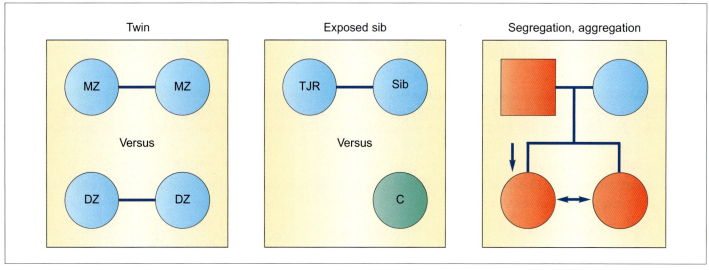

1.14 Strategies to determine the genetic contribution to osteoarthritis. Classic twin studies (left) compare the concordance for osteoarthritis in monozygotic (MZ) (identical) and dizygotic (DZ) (non-identical) twins – a higher concordance in monozygotic twins suggests genetic predisposition.

A higher prevalence of osteoarthritis (middle), compared to controls (C), in siblings (Sib) of patients with hip or knee osteoarthritis severe enough to lead to joint replacement (TJR) also suggests genetic predisposition to osteoarthritis.

Examination of the way osteoarthritis transmits vertically and horizontally through families (right), compared to the expected population prevalence of osteoarthritis, can show familial clustering.

1.15 Two sisters affected by nodal generalized osteoarthritis affecting hands and knees. A sibling of someone who has required joint replacement for knee osteoarthritis is at more than twice the risk of developing knee osteoarthritis than someone without such a 'genetic exposure'; the risk for a sibling of someone who has undergone joint replacement for hip osteoarthritis is even higher (3–9 fold depending on age and gender). Genetic studies undertaken on multiples families with such affected sibling pairs is the main way of determining linkage between osteoarthritis and specific chromosomal regions. Examination of possible candidate genes within those regions is a common strategy to determine the genes responsible for genetic susceptibility.

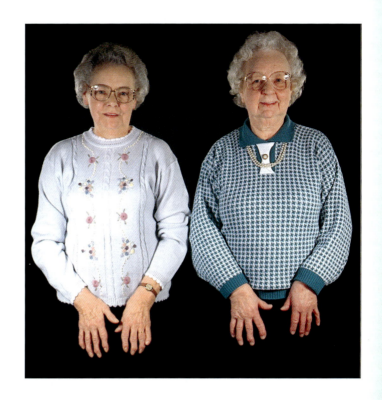

1.16 Diagram showing osteoarthritis to be a 'common complex disorder'. Multiple (currently unknown) polymorphisms need to interact with other constitutional or local risk factors to permit expression of the osteoarthritis phenotype. These risk factors may vary according to joint site. Risk factors for development of osteoarthritis may also differ from risk factors for a good or bad clinical outcome. Blue shading represents commonly affected joints.

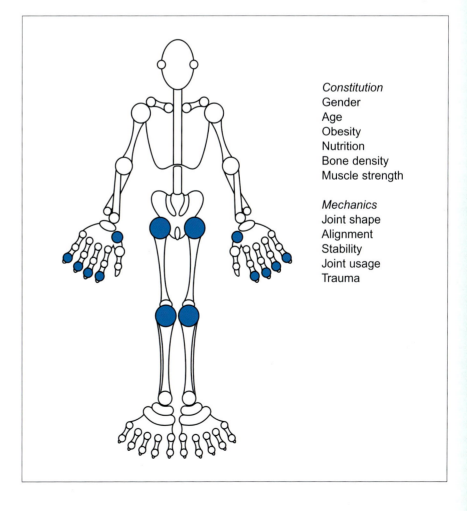

Constitution
Gender
Age
Obesity
Nutrition
Bone density
Muscle strength

Mechanics
Joint shape
Alignment
Stability
Joint usage
Trauma

Occupation

A role for occupation in the development of osteoarthritis is often cited by patients, and can be an important discussion point in medico–legal claims. Early studies of mill and cotton workers from the UK and USA suggested that differing occupational hand usage could influence the pattern and distribution of osteoarthritis in the hand. What was not clear from these studies was whether there was an absolute increase in the prevalence of osteoarthritis or simply a different localization of disease. A similar argument is often debated for trauma – does trauma increase the risk or does it just bring forward the development of osteoarthritis in patients at risk?

In at least one occupation, that is, farming, an increased risk of hip osteoarthritis has been demonstrated compared to appropriate controls. This risk appears greatest for arable farmers and for farmers brought up as children on a farm, but the precise mechanism is unclear. Because the risk is more than twofold, UK farmers who develop hip osteoarthritis are entitled to industrial compensation.

In many cases, simple job descriptions do not adequately describe the actual locomotor stresses that are involved. Accordingly, attempts have been made to examine and quantify the actual amount of a particular activity that an occupation involves, and to examine these as risk factors for osteoarthritis. Using such an approach, it has been demonstrated that repeated occupational knee bending, particularly if this involves heavy lifting, associates with an increased risk of knee osteoarthritis.

Sport

The role of sport in the development of osteoarthritis is not entirely clear. Moderate levels of sporting activity appear to improve functional outcome in osteoarthritis. This may be mediated by the benefits to neuromuscular functioning, improved aerobic fitness and well-being, easier weight control, and improved self-efficacy. Even at elite levels, overall, participation in sport appears to be beneficial. However, pitted against this is the risk of trauma from direct injury or from more minor trauma that is repetitive and still bad for joint health. Therefore, it seems likely that exercise/activity and osteoarthritis will show a U-shaped, rather than linear, dose–response relationship (**1.17**).

Despite the overall benefits of exercise, moderate–elite sporting activity appears to increase osteophyte formation though this may not be true osteophyte (that associates with cartilage loss) but rather a stress reaction at entheseal insertions. Power lifting has been associated with knee osteoarthritis, presumably sharing the same biomechanical mechanism as with occupational knee bending. Other sports, such as football, are associated with osteoarthritis, but it is suspected that much of this is related to direct trauma and a high prevalence of internal derangement and instability. More minor but repetitive trauma may be injurious, and different patterns of osteoarthritis have been reported in different types of sports, leading to specific terms such as: mid-tarsal arthritis – footballers; 'pitchers elbow' – baseball; and ballerina's foot.

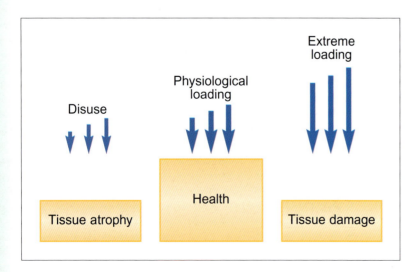

1.17 Joints are designed to move. Under-usage leads to tissue atrophy and is bad for joint health. Excessive activity may lead to tissue injury and predispose to osteoarthritis. Moderate, regular activity that provides physiological loading without tissue injury seems the ideal between these two extremes.

Muscle

The synovial joint does not simply involve cartilage, synovial lining, fluid, and bone: it is a complex organ that requires many other tissues for successful function. Amongst these is muscle (**1.18**). Often overlooked in early studies, a renewed interest occurred when it was demonstrated that muscle weakness is very prominent in patients with knee osteoarthritis. Indeed, studies from Bristol and elsewhere demonstrated very clearly that muscle weakness was a more important associate of disability than the degree of structural change as evidenced by radiography. Apart from its role as a prime mover of joints, muscle is an important proprioceptive organ, and muscle weakness related to knee osteoarthritis also associates with reduced knee proprioception, increased sway when standing with eyes shut, an increased risk of falls, and an abnormal gait pattern.

Experimental models confirm that arthropathy can rapidly produce marked weakness of adjacent muscles. This results from a combination of neural inhibition of muscle activation and an increased, but imbalanced, turnover of muscle tissue resulting in muscle atrophy. This observation has important therapeutic implications, as will be discussed later (page 97).

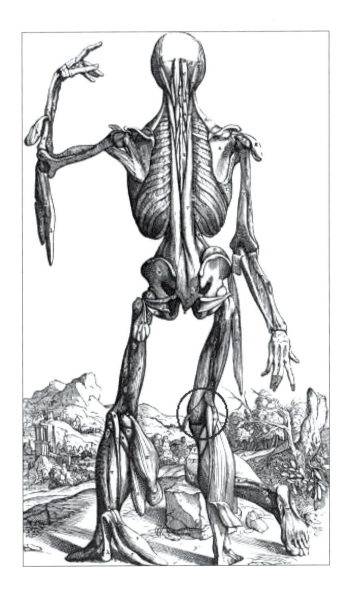

1.18 Muscles are essential for normal joint function (from the second book of *De Humani Corporis Fabrica* [1543], by Andreus Vesalius [1514–1568]).

Neurological factors

If muscles are important in osteoarthritis, then it is likely that neurological factors may also be important. It is clear that the muscle weakness and atrophy observed are critically dependent on neurological function. In animals with experimental acute knee damage, muscle atrophy is critically dependent upon on an intact dorsal root ganglion and reflex arc. Similarly, in a number of different forms of osteoarthritis, the presence of pre-existent or subsequent neurological disease can markedly affect the phenotypic expression of arthritis (**1.19**).

This clinical observation has had clinical correlates in various animal models of osteoarthritis, including in the guinea pig and the dog. More recently, it has been suggested that neurological dysfunction may play a role in the initiation of osteoarthritis in man. In a study of young, asymptomatic adults suspected to be at high risk of the subsequent development of knee osteoarthritis, subtle abnormalities in neuromuscular 'bracing' have been measured, and referred to as 'micro-klutziness'. This may simply reflect a protopathic bias, that is, the presence of pre-clinical disease. However, examination of the relatives of these affected individuals suggests that this phenomenon might predate development of any pathology.

Other joint and bone disease

Other disorders of joints may predispose to subsequent osteoarthritis. These include other defined arthropathies, such as rheumatoid arthritis, psoriatic arthritis, sepsis, juvenile idiopathic arthritis, and gout. This does not usually present a diagnostic difficulty, but it is important to consider since supervening osteoarthritis may require a very different therapeutic approach to the underlying inflammatory joint disease. With primary inflammatory arthritis such as rheumatoid, it is usually only when the inflammatory, damaging synovitis is controlled that any attempts at tissue repair can occur and 'secondary' osteoarthritis can develop.

Childhood disorders, such as Perthe's disease, slipped femoral epiphysis, or mild acetabular dysplasia (**1.20**) at the hip may compromise the joint, and if untreated predispose to osteoarthritis in the adult.

Similarly, disorders of adjacent bone (Paget's disease, for example) may also be associated with osteoarthritis. This may occur because of adverse effects on cartilage and bone that accompany bone remodelling and altered bone vascularity (**1.21**).

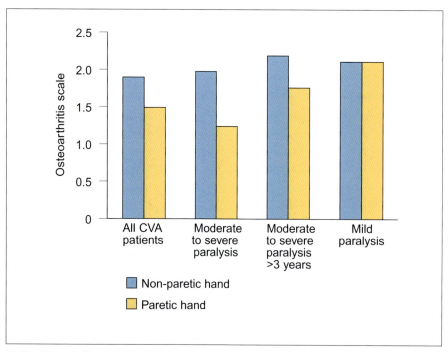

1.19 Effect of a stroke on the subsequent development of osteoarthritis. (Data derived from Segal R, Avrahami E, Lebdinski E, *et al.* [1998]. The impact of hemiparalysis on the expression of osteoarthritis. *Arthritis Rheum*, **41**:2249–2256.)

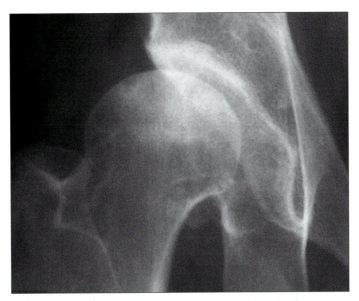

1.20 A shallow acetabular roof, as seen here in the context of minor acetabular dysplasia, can allow the femoral head to migrate upwards and outwards and lead to osteoarthritis.

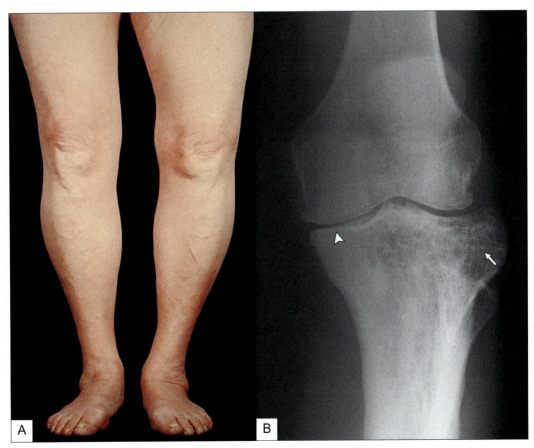

1.21 Paget's disease causing bowing of the left tibia (**A**). The x-ray (**B**) shows the abnormal Pagetic bone abutting up to the knee (arrow), widening of the tibia which no longer matches the femoral width, and associated cartilage loss (arrowhead) in both tibiofemoral compartments. Cartilage loss is often more extensive and diffuse with such 'Pagetic arthropathy' than with common osteoarthritis.

Genetically determined conditions that affect bone or cartilage may result in premature 'osteoarthritis' at multiple sites, sometimes in association with short stature, body disproportion, and other clinical features. The most common of these conditions are the many forms of multiple epiphyseal dysplasia (1.22–1.24). When the spine is involved, it is called spondyloepiphyseal dysplasia. A family history may sometimes be present, but in many cases it appears to result from an apparently spontaneous mutation. Radiographic appearances are often characteristic.

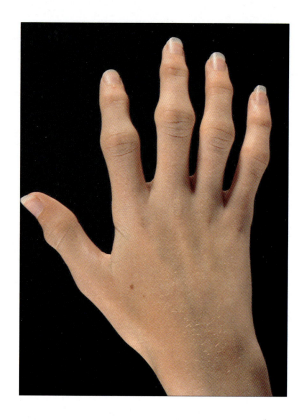

1.22 Hand of a 24-year-old woman with spondyloepiphyseal dysplasia showing what clinically appears to be osteoarthritis of multiple interphalangeal joints characterized by bony swelling.

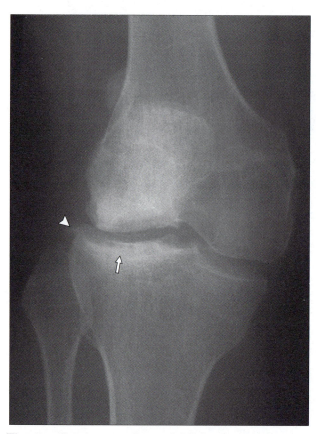

1.23 The standing knee radiograph of the same patient as **1.22**. Note the abnormal tilt of the tibiofemoral joint line and the sclerosis (arrow) and osteophyte (arrowhead) that mainly involves the lateral compartment.

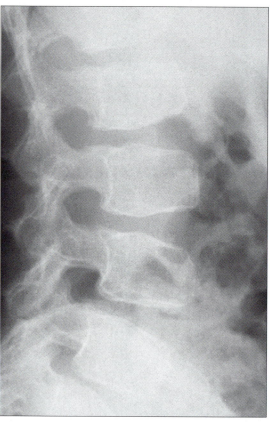

1.24 The lumbar spine radiograph of the same patient showing anterior-posterior elongation of the vertebral bodies, the abnormal contours to the endplates, and the widening of the anterior disc spaces.

Toxins and metabolic factors

Geographical 'hot-spots' of endemic osteoarthritis have been recognized for some time. Perhaps the best characterized of these is Kashin–Beck disease. This presents as a premature form of polyarticular osteoarthritis in Mongolia, eastern Russia and northern China. Other similar forms are often named according to the area or population affected, e.g. Mselini disease in southern Africa, and Malmad disease in India. Early studies involving migration of people into and out of the affected regions suggested environmental, rather than genetic factors in its pathogenesis. Recent studies have started to identify some of those factors. For example, Kashin–Beck disease almost certainly results from an interaction between selenium deficiency and hypothyroidism due to iodine deficiency, that appears to encourage chondrocyte death in hyaline cartilage of children and young adults. While these endemic arthropathies are clearly dissimilar from sporadic osteoarthritis and present at a very young age (2nd and 3rd decades), they suggest the possibility that other toxins and metabolic factors may be important in the development of more common 'sporadic' osteoarthritis.

Haemochromatosis is an increasingly well-understood genetic disorder where there is a marked accumulation of iron in tissues, including the joint. There is a clearly-defined arthropathy of haemochromatosis which is very similar to osteoarthritis, notably the subset known as pyrophosphate arthropathy (page 44). The mechanism by which arthropathy is produced is not completely defined, but there is an accumulation of iron within cartilage and synovium, which may cause direct toxicity to chondrocytes. The observed arthropathy often involves aggressive loss of joint space at sites (such as the metacarpophalangeal joints, and radiocarpal joint), that are less commonly affected in sporadic osteoarthritis (**1.25–1.27**). Multiple subchondral cysts are a prominent feature. In addition, iron interferes with inorganic pyrophosphate metabolism, and leads to increased production and crystallization of calcium pyrophosphate crystals. This may be observed radiographically as chondrocalcinosis, and clinically as acute crystal synovitis.

Acromegaly also associates with an arthropathy that clinically and radiographically resembles osteoarthritis. The mechanism is unclear, but interestingly there is often initial widening of the joint space (**1.28**). Pathologically, there is an exuberant thickening of the hyaline cartilage, but this outgrows the nutrient supply provided below by the bone

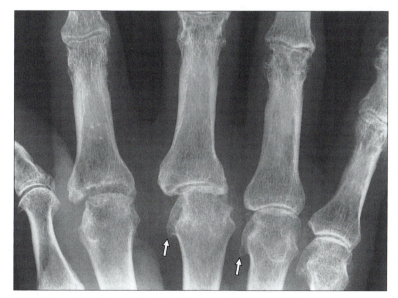

1.25 Hand radiograph of a 56-year-old man with haemochromatosis showing eccentric joint space loss and hook osteophytes (arrows) on the radial aspect of the metacarpal heads. Symptomatic arthritis was the presenting feature of his haemochromatosis.

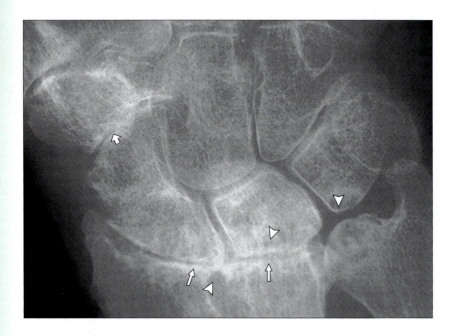

1.26 The wrist radiograph of the same patient as in **1.25**, showing cartilage loss in the 1st carpometacarpal and trapezio-scaphoid joints (short arrow) (common sites for osteoarthritis), but also in the radiocarpal (arrows) and midcarpal rows (sites not usually affected by osteoarthritis). Multiple subchondral cysts are a prominent feature in the radiocarpal joint (arrowheads).

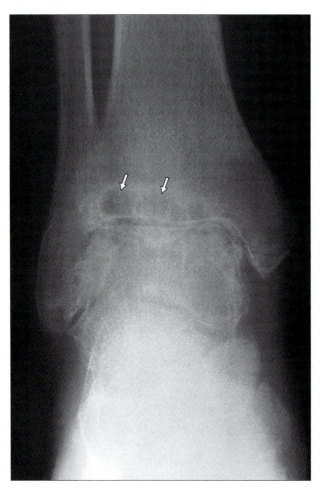

1.27 The ankle radiograph of the same patient as **1.26**, showing marked cartilage loss and again multiple cysts (arrows).

blood vessels and superficially by the synovial fluid. Subsequently, there is erosion and loss of the cartilage and eventual joint space narrowing. In addition, there may be alteration of the bones with periosteal, cortical thickening.

Avascular necrosis (osteonecrosis) can result in collapse and involution of a segment of bone and its overlying cartilage. The subsequent distortion of the anatomical shape of the joint then results in osteoarthritis. Avascular necrosis may be secondary to conditions that cause external compression of blood vessels in bone (e.g. steroid therapy, and alcohol excess – mainly due to increased fat deposition in bone) or reduced intravascular flow (e.g. sickle cell anaemia, and Caisson's disease – the 'bends'). In these situations, it mainly targets the hip (femoral head, **1.29**) shoulder (humeral head), knee (distal femur), or elbow (distal humerus). Primary osteonecrosis of large bones usually targets the medial femoral condyle (**1.30**). Osteochondritis, resulting from trauma during childhood or developmental abnormality, affects small bones and may be a predisposing factor to subsequent osteoarthritis (e.g. osteonecrosis of the lunate – Kienbock's disease).

Although relatively uncommon, presentation of what clinically appears to be osteoarthritis at a young age (under 55), or in an atypical pattern, or both, should lead to consideration of an underlying disease. The usual cause of young onset osteoarthritis at a single joint site is preceding trauma, and this is often apparent in the patient's history or on the x-ray. However, for young onset osteoarthritis affecting several or multiple joints, several conditions may require consideration (*Table 1.2*).

1.28 Standing knee radiographs of a 52-year-old man with acromegaly who presented with arthralgia, and symptoms and signs of osteoarthritis in his hands. His knees show obvious widening of the tibiofemoral joint spaces and bony enlargement ('squaring') of the femoral condyles.

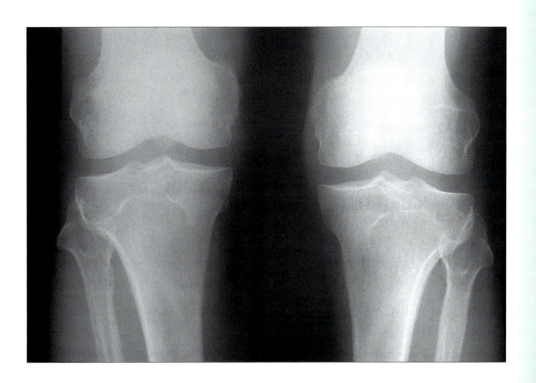

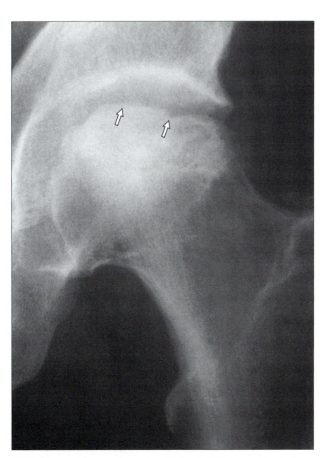

1.29 Late osteonecrosis of the left femoral head in a 39-year-old patient who had received high dose steroids for asthma, showing segmental collapse and increased sclerosis of the superior pole (arrows).

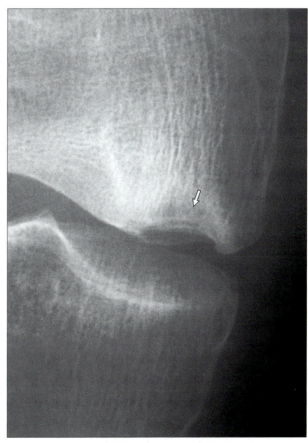

1.30 Idiopathic medial femoral necrosis showing localized segmental collapse, sclerosis, and altered contour of the distal femur (arrow).

Table 1.2 Causes of young-onset osteoarthritis or osteoarthritis with atypical distribution

Monoarticular
- Prior trauma
- Localized instability
- Avascular necrosis

Pauci/polyarticular
- Prior joint disease (e.g. juvenile idiopathic arthritis)
- Spondyloepiphyseal dysplasia
- Metabolic disease – haemochromatosis
- Endocrine disease – acromegaly
- Avascular necrosis
- Neuropathic (Charcot) joint
- Endemic osteoarthritis

Mortality and co-morbidity in osteoarthritis

Osteoarthritis is not an entirely benign disease, in terms of general health. A number of studies have demonstrated an increased mortality in osteoarthritis, although the cause for this unclear. Although this a small relative risk, the attributable population risk is high because of the high prevalence of osteoarthritis.

A number of co-morbidities principally associated with obesity and insulin resistance ('metabolic syndrome') are also associated with osteoarthritis. These include: diabetes, hypertension, cardiovascular disease, and gout. In dealing with patients with osteoarthritis, it is important to consider these issues.

Towards a definition of osteoarthritis

One of the problems that has bedevilled the study of osteoarthritis is that while clinicians instinctively recognize when a patient has osteoarthritis, defining it in a form which is easily communicated to others has proved more difficult. Clearly, the reason for defining osteoarthritis may affect how it is defined. For example, if the purpose is to look at determinants of structural change, then a radiographic or pathologic definition may be required. However, if the purpose is to define patients who may be suitable for a clinical trial, then the only appropriate ones are those with symptoms which also may demonstrate structural (radiographic) change. Even if structural change and symptoms can be agreed upon, some form of grading of severity may be important and, indeed, individual aspects may require separate evaluation.

Pathological features

Pathological changes are central to many definitions of osteoarthritis. In essence, an osteoarthritic joint has changes in many, if not all, of its tissue components.

The most obvious change is in the articular hyaline cartilage. The earliest change is thought to be increased hydration followed by softening and fissuring of the surface. Eventually, this results in thinning of the cartilage and exposure of the subchondral bone (**1.31**). These changes are focal, and generally occur mainly at sites of maximum mechanical stress within the joint.

Changes in bone are also prominent (**1.32, 1.33**). At the macroscopic level, this involves thickening of the subchondral bone (apparent as sclerosis) and formation of osteophyte. The formation of osteophyte is initiated by new fibrocartilage that subsequently undergoes endochondral ossification, usually at the joint margins at sites of capsule and ligament insertions. Small areas of pressure damage and osteonecrosis may also result in loss of bone. At the microscopic level, avascular necrosis is probably a more common mechanism than is generally appreciated. Holes or 'cysts' may also occur in bone (**1.32**) some of which communicate with the joint cavity. These most likely reflect liquefaction following localized osteonecrosis, or possibly arise at sites where synovial fluid is forced under pressure through clefts in the cartilage and subchondral bone.

But osteoarthritis is not just about hyaline cartilage and bone. The synovium in osteoarthritis may show marked inflammation, though this is patchy rather than diffuse, as in inflammatory rheumatoid disease. The mechanism underlying this is far from being understood. It may represent secondary 'debris synovitis', with the synovium being inflamed by small shards of cartilage and bone that become free within the damaged joint (**1.33**). Another possible cause of inflammation could be due to calcium pyrophosphate and

1.31 Macroscopic appearance of tibia removed during joint replacement for osteoarthritis. Note the unequal, and in this case, severe loss of articular cartilage with antero-posterior grooves in the exposed subchondral bone of the medial tibial plateau (arrow). Note also the florid rolling osteophyte at the joint margins.

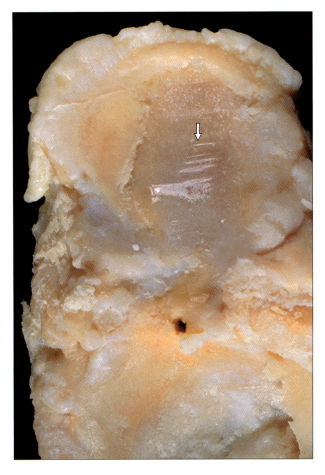

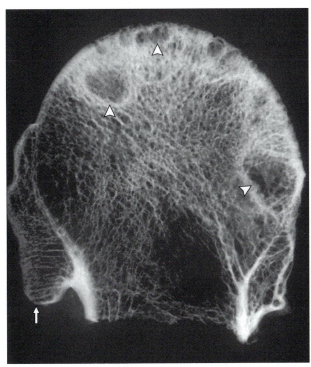

1.32 Slab radiograph of an osteoarthritic femoral head showing florid marginal osteophyte (arrow) and multiple small and large 'cysts' with sclerotic borders (arrowheads).

1.33 Small fragments of cartilage within synovial fluid from an osteoarthritic knee (x400 magnification). These fragments may be taken up by synoviocytes and cause local inflammation.

apatite crystals released from osteoarthritic cartilage (**1.34**). A low-grade primary inflammatory process may, however, underlie some cases. As a result osteoarthritic synovium can be thickened, have an infiltrate of inflammatory cells, and show a marked degree of vascularity.

Intra-articular fibrocartilage (e.g. in the knee menisci), is commonly affected in osteoarthritis, showing the same histological changes, thinning, and fibrillation as hyaline cartilage (**1.35**). It may reflect the generalized nature of the osteoarthritis process, or the altered biomechanics within the joint. Alternatively, meniscal injury may predate the osteoarthritis, and be a predisposing risk factor. Although post-meniscectomy osteoarthritis has long been recognized, recent MRI studies suggest that meniscal abnormality may be a very common feature of early osteoarthritis.

Ligaments and tendons also demonstrate degenerative changes with thinning and weakening. Again, and quite interestingly, MRI studies have suggested that this may be an early feature of osteoarthritis and, perhaps in some situations, predate cartilage and bone disease.

Neuromuscular changes are also commonly seen with atrophy and increased muscle turnover, as well as increased innervation in conjunction with angiogenesis.

Definition of presence of osteoarthritis

For many studies and, indeed, often in the clinical setting, the establishment of the presence or absence of osteoarthritis is all that is required. However, not all structural osteoarthritis is symptomatic. The correlation between presence of osteoarthritis and the occurrence of associated pain and disability varies between joint sites, and in general is not strong (**1.36**). Most certainly, at a number of sites asymptomatic osteoarthritis is far more common than symptomatic change.

The most common symptom of osteoarthritis, and the one that most concerns patients, is pain. While it would seem that the presence or absence of pain at a specific location would be easy to establish, in fact, even subtle differences in the wording of the question(s) used can result in major differences in the prevalence of osteoarthritis. Furthermore, the localization of pain at different joint sites can sometimes prove problematic. For example, in the spine pain can commonly radiate widely and may arise from a number of other structures and sites. Sometimes it is very to difficult to establish whether apparent radiographic osteoarthritis is symptomatic or not.

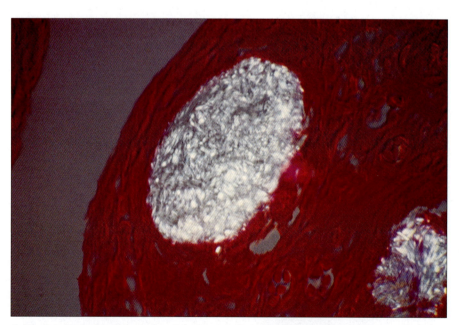

1.34 Large collections of calcium pyrophosphate crystals within osteoarthritic synovium (x200 magnification). These inflammatory crystals form in hyaline and fibro-cartilage, but may then be shed into the joint cavity and be taken up by synovium, resulting in synovitis.

1.35 Degeneration and tearing of a meniscus in an osteoarthric knee removed at joint replacement. Note the severe fibrillation and thinning of the hyaline cartilage of the underlying tibial plateau.

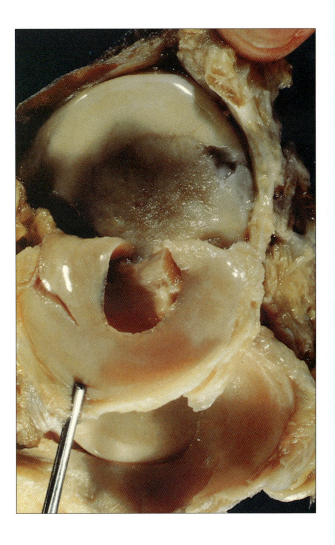

1.36 Diagram showing the imprecise inter-relationship between the presence of pain, disability and structural change of osteoarthritis. The correlation is best at the hip, but is generally poor at other sites (especially the spine and hand).

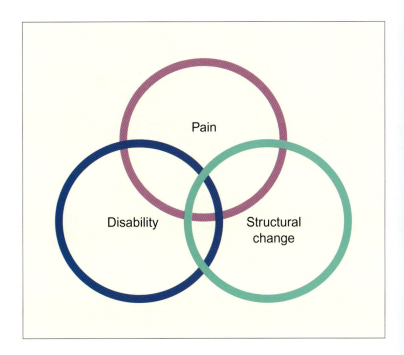

Regional pain in relation to osteoarthritis can arise for a number of reasons (**1.37**). There are no clear differences in the characteristics of osteoarthritic pain that distinguish it from other causes of pain. Thus whether symptoms can be used as a reliable surrogate for osteoarthritis in the absence of some form of structural assessment would seem unlikely.

Conversely, whether radiographic or other structural definitions alone can be used to define osteoarthritis is equally problematic if the purpose of the definition is to define the clinical problem.

Finally, clinical signs can be used in various combinations with structural and symptomatic change to define osteoarthritis. Unfortunately, the major problem with this is that all studies that have examined the reliability and reproducibility of clinical signs have suggested that many of these, with the possible exception of Heberden's nodes, can be very unreliable. In addition, their relationship to underlying radiographic change can be problematic.

Currently, radiographic osteoarthritis is usually defined by the presence of a definite osteophyte on an appropriate radiograph, especially for knee and hand osteoarthritis, or by definite focal joint space narrowing (the main feature used for hip osteoarthritis).

Symptomatic osteoarthritis can be defined in a number of ways. One example of this is the American College of Rheumatology (ACR) definition of knee osteoarthritis (*Table 1.3*). Using this system the best definition requires the presence of pain and either a radiographic, clinical feature (crepitus), or demographic feature (age >50 years). However, this demonstrates the problem with adopting a universal definition. The ACR definition was created and developed in order to differentiate between patients with symptomatic knee osteoarthritis and those with inflammatory arthritis in a rheumatology service setting. As such, it is appropriate in defining a population drawn from a hospital base suitable for clinical trials in osteoarthritis, but perhaps not in defining osteoarthritis for epidemiological purposes or community service settings where radiographs may be impractical. It also does not address the issue of asymptomatic radiographic change, nor the fact that the detection of clinical signs is insensitive and unreliable, and the defined age cut-off may miss early disease. Definition thus remains problematic.

Assessing symptoms in osteoarthritis

There are various symptoms that are associated with osteoarthritis (*Table 1.4*). Of these, pain is the most clinically relevant. Pain itself can be subdivided into various categories according to its timing (usage pain, rest pain, and night pain). There is some evidence that this may have clinical relevance with, for example, pain at rest, and at night being more responsive to NSAIDs than to acetaminophen (paracetamol). Pain in osteoarthritis tends to be worse towards the end of the day. It also shows a weekly (circaseptan) variation in being worse around the weekend, even in people who are not working (**1.38**).

Table 1.3 ACR criteria for knee osteoarthritis

Knee pain (majority of previous month)	*Knee pain (majority of previous month)*
	X-ray with osteophyte
Plus three of the following:	Plus one of the following:
• Age >50 years	• Age >50 years
• Morning stiffness <30 minutes	• Morning stiffness <30 minutes
• Crepitus	• Crepitus
• Bony enlargement on palpation	
• Bony tenderness	
• No palpable warmth	

1.37 Osteoarthritis may give rise to pain from intraosseous hypertension and microfracture (yellow), intracapsular hypertension (synovial thickening, increased fluid production, capsular tightening) (green), or from periarticular syndromes, such as bursitis, tendinitis, and enthesopathy (red), secondary to remodelling and altered joint mechanics.

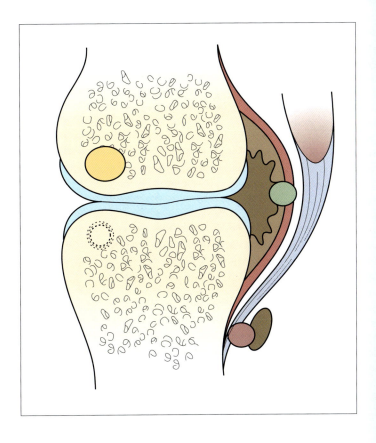

Table 1.4 Symptoms associated with osteoarthritis

Pain:
- on movement
- at night
- at rest

Stiffness

Deformity

Loss of range of movement

Crepitus

Locking

Giving way

Muscle weakness and wasting

Nerve compression (spine)

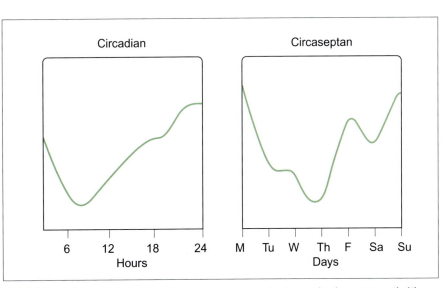

1.38 Circadian and circaseptan variation in pain intensity in osteoarthritis. (Adapted from Bellamy N, Sothern RB, Campbell J [1990]. Rhythmic variations in pain perception in osteoarthritis of the knee. *J Rheumatol*, **17**:364–372.)

Stiffness – a subjective feeling of difficulty in moving – also occurs in osteoarthritis. Usually it is relatively brief (5–10 minutes) and rarely lasts more than 30 minutes either in the morning (morning stiffness) or after rest ('gelling').

Some patients complain of crepitus, which is a rough palpable or occasionally audible vibration on movement. Although this is sometimes assessed by examination, this sign is unreliable and grading systems are not used.

Deformity, either in terms of bony swelling or malalignment across the joint, is common, but is rarely subject to measurement or grading.

Muscle wasting around affected joints is common. Measurement of both muscle size (girth and imaging) and muscle function (strength and power) can be performed, and may be used to assess disease progress.

Various composite measures have been developed in order to assess and score pain and functional impairment in osteoarthritis. Perhaps the two best developed and used measures are the Western Ontario and McMasters Universities (WOMAC) Osteoarthritis Index and the Lesquesne Algofunctional Index. The scores derived by these disease-specific instruments can be separated into their specific domains (pain, stiffness, and function), or used as a single composite score.

Assessing structural (radiographic) change in osteoarthritis

Radiographs can be used to detect the presence or absence of osteoarthritis, and to assess progression of structural change. Plain radiographs are the traditional imaging measure, and they are easy to obtain and readily available. Radiographic features of osteoarthritis include focal joint space narrowing (from cartilage thinning), marginal osteophyte, sclerosis (increased whiteness of subchondral bone), bone cysts and osteochondral 'loose' bodies, and eventually bone attrition, deformity of bone ends, and malalignment (**1.39**).

The most widely used system to analyse and grade radiographic osteoarthritis is the Kellgren and Lawrence composite system (*Table 1.5*). This employs combined assessment of individual features, and can be scored using the verbal descriptions or by comparison with a standard radiographic atlas. There are problems with the system, as the hierarchy of change may not be as described, standardization may be problematic, and radiographs are by definition two-dimensional and may thus underestimate the degree of involvement. It does, however, provide a method for categorizing joint involvement into four or five simple grades.

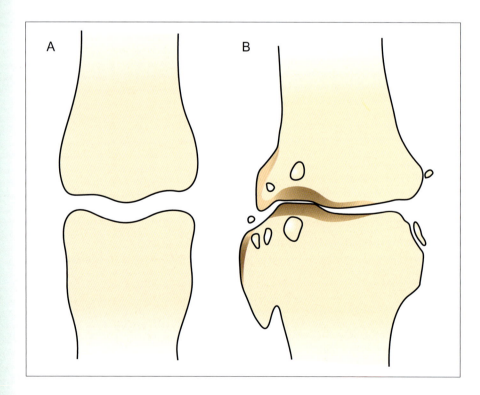

1.39 Diagram showing a normal joint outline (**A**) and the major features of osteoarthritis (**B**). These include focal joint space narrowing, marginal osteophyte, subchondral sclerosis, cysts, osteochondral bodies and eventual deformity of bone ends, and malalignment.

The problems with the system have led to attempts to develop other ways of assessing radiographs for osteoarthritic changes. Generally, these have involved the development of atlases of standard images and the separate grading of individual features (osteophyte, joint space narrowing, etc.). One system for knee osteoarthritis that uses line drawings rather than photographs has a number of advantages, including: an interval rather than ordinal scale for narrowing and osteophyte; a value for normal joint space width that is based on a population sample; separate images for narrowing and osteophyte (thus avoiding the distraction and bias when several features occur together); uniform magnification of images; and separate atlases for joint space narrowing for men and women (men have wider joint spaces at the knee) (**1.40**).

Since cartilage loss is often considered the major feature of osteoarthritis and joint space loss the major surrogate for this, then it makes sense to try to quantify this accurately. Standardization of radiographic technique is clearly important as an initial step, and several methods are available to increase reproducibility and precision of radiographs. This has been combined with various measurement techniques (both manual and semi- or fully-automated) to achieve this.

Several important consequences of these approaches have emerged. The joint space widths in women and men at different ages have been defined. For the hip, at least, a definition has been established of hip osteoarthritis based on the level of joint space width which best correlates with the presence or absence of symptoms.

As regards the specific features of osteoarthritis, their individual association with symptoms varies and, thus, their usefulness in defining osteoarthritis. For example, at the hip it is joint space narrowing, not osteophyte, that most closely associates with hip pain. Conversely, at the knee it is osteophyte, not narrowing, that associates best with knee pain, such that even quite minor osteophytosis is a reasonable correlate of symptomatic osteoarthritis. However, in assessing disease progression at the knee, joint space measurement is more accurate and sensitive to change than grading of osteophyte. One possible problem at the knee is that pain can affect loading of the joint and hence measured joint space width. This has been postulated as a mechanism to explain how symptom-modifying drugs may falsely appear to associate with slowing or even reversal of joint space narrowing. The maximally-thinned cartilage in the tibiofemoral compartments is brought into the weight-bearing position when the knee is semi-flexed. If pain is relieved, the knees often straighten more, thus bringing wider, less-affected cartilage into the weight-bearing position, and making the radiographic joint space appear wider than before.

Table 1.5 Kellgren and Lawrence grading system for osteoarthritis

Grade 0	Normal
Grade 1	Doubtful narrowing of joint space, possible osteophyte
Grade 2	Definite osteophyte, possible narrowing
Grade 3	Moderate multiple osteophytes, definite narrowing, some sclerosis, possible deformity of bone ends
Grade 4	Large osteophytes, marked narrowing, severe sclerosis, definite deformity of bone ends

(Adapted from *The Epidemiology of Chronic Rheumatism. Volume II Atlas of Standard Radiographs of Arthritis*, Blackwell Scientific Publications [1963].)

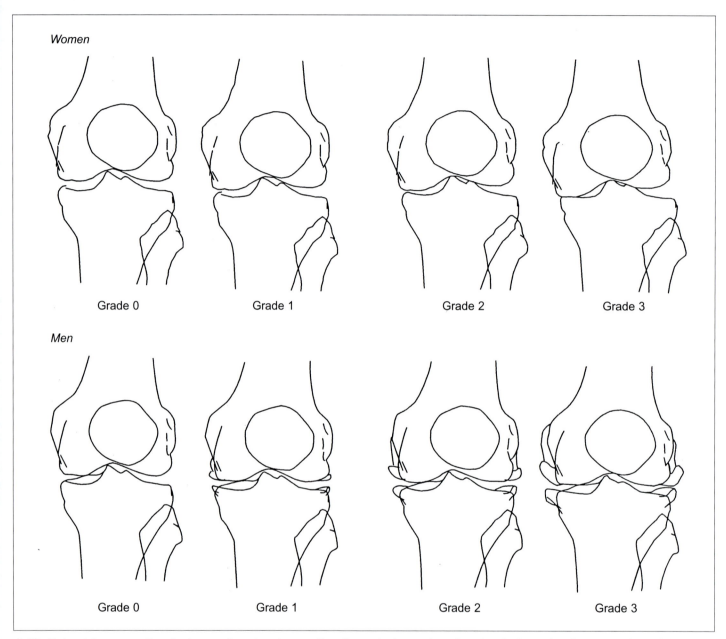

1.40 Extract from an atlas that uses line drawings rather than photographs, showing 0–3 grades for narrowing of the medial tibiofemoral compartment in women (top row) and 0–3 grades for osteophyte at all tibiofemoral sites. (From Nagaosa Y, Mateus M, Hassan B, *et al*. [2000]. Development of a logically devised line drawing atlas for grading of knee osteoarthritis. *Ann Rheum Dis*, **59**:587–595.)

Is osteoarthritis useful?

The fact that osteoarthritis has been observed in many species and throughout evolutionary time has led to speculation that it has been conserved for a reason, that is, it may have a selection advantage. Of course, this may simply reflect the fact that osteoarthritis in humans is a disease of older, non-reproductive age so there is no negative selection pressure which would confer a survival disadvantage, but it does not explain its presence in other species. However, one perspective is that this so-called 'degenerative disease' is the inherent repair process of synovial joints that in some circumstances may confer survival advantage. As has been alluded to before, it could be argued that osteoarthritis is essentially a reparative process, characterized by new tissue production (especially bone) that is brought into action by a variety of joint insults (**1.41**). In general, it is an efficient repair process, and often compensates for the triggering insult without associating with symptoms or disability. Osteophytosis and bone remodelling may increase the surface area of the compromised joint and beneficially redistribute load transmission, and vertically growing osteophyes may splint the joint and counter instability. In this sense, the osteoarthritic response can be seen as potentially beneficial.

It is only if osteoarthritis cannot compensate due to overwhelming insult or a poor repair response that 'decompensated' osteoarthritis may associate with pain and disability and become a clinical problem. Such a scenario explains the marked clinical heterogeneity of osteoarthritis, the high prevalence of asymptomatic osteoarthritis, and the often good outcome of symptomatic cases. Decompensated symptomatic osteoarthritis may be seen as a form of end-stage 'joint failure' with a common phenotype irrespective of the triggering insult.

Further reading

Brandt KD, Doherty M, Lohmander LS (2003). *Osteoarthritis*, 2nd edn, Oxford University Press, Oxford.

Felson DT (Conference Chair) (2000). Osteoarthritis: New Insights Part 1. The disease and its risk factors. *Ann Intern Med*, **133**:635–649.

Moskowitz RW, Howell DS, Altman RD, *et al.* (2001). *Osteoarthritis: Diagnosis and Medical/Surgical Management.* WB Saunders, London.

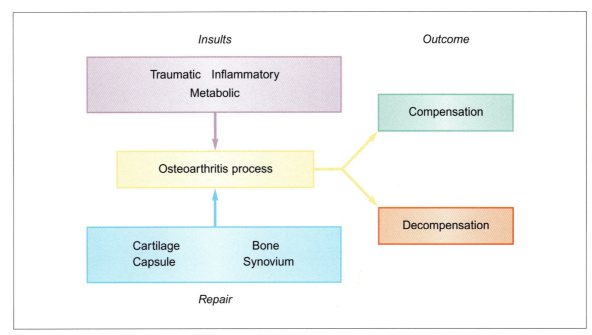

1.41 The proposed scenario of osteoarthritis as the inherent repair process of synovial joints. It is only if this slow, efficient repair process cannot compensate for the triggering insults that the joint continues to remodel and more commonly associates with symptoms and disability.

Chapter 2

General features of osteoarthritis

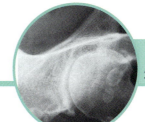

What are the clinical features of osteoarthritis?

The clinical features of osteoarthritis relate to both symptoms and signs. As has been discussed in Chapter 1, the principle symptom of osteoarthritis is pain. Typically this occurs during movement and/or loading of the joint. It may vary greatly in severity from mild to very severe. Indeed, as already discussed, structural change may be entirely asymptomatic. Usually pain from osteoarthritis changes only slowly and undergoes variation with 'good weeks' and 'bad weeks'. Some authors consider that osteoarthritis undergoes 'flares' with temporary marked increases in pain and swelling, although the mechanism underlying this is unclear.

Nocturnal pain may be a prominent feature. Although taken as a late, poor prognostic feature by some, it may be present early in the clinical course, and possibly may be particularly helped by NSAIDs. The mechanism in this situation is thought to be vascular in nature with increased intraosseous pressure. As was discussed earlier, this can be associated with localized areas of avascular necrosis and more rapid deterioration in joint architecture with more rapid clinical progression.

Osteophyte growth and bony remodelling can result in altered joint shape and, at superficial sites, this can readily be observed clinically (**2.1**). Similarly, loss of bone stock, often as a result of avascular necrosis, may result in malalignment with resultant varus, valgus, flexion, or other deformities (**2.2**). Again these deformities can be readily observed, and may be a risk factor for future progression and deterioration.

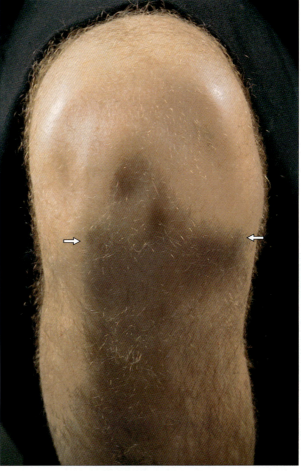

2.1 Femoral osteophyte is visible and palpable in this flexed knee as prominent bony ridging (arrows) along the anterior border of each condyle giving an inverted 'V' appearance.

Swelling that is due to soft-tissue rather than bony enlargement may be observed. Although synovial thickening may be a factor, it is more commonly due to increased synovial fluid and distension of the joint capsule. Joint swellings due to fluid tend to occur in natural weak areas of the capsule, and thus in characteristic locations. Acute swellings may sometimes occur in a fashion similar to that seen in the 'flares' of pain. The mechanism is again unclear, although in some cases a crystal synovitis may occur, most commonly related to calcium pyrophosphate crystals ('pseudogout') (2.3).

In association with crystal synovitis, an overlying erythema may occur, but in general cutaneous features including local heat are unusual.

Stiffness in osteoarthritis is usually relatively short-lived and often more related to inactivity, such as sitting, rather than being the more typical and very prolonged early morning stiffness seen in, for example, rheumatoid arthritis.

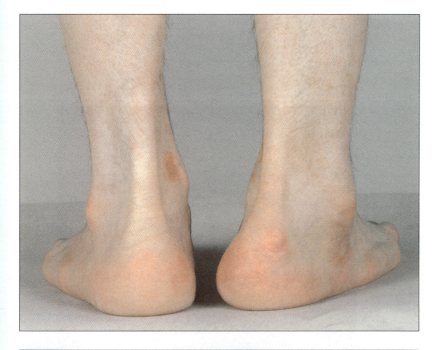

2.2 Right hindfoot varus deformity in a patient with chronic pyrophosphate arthropathy.

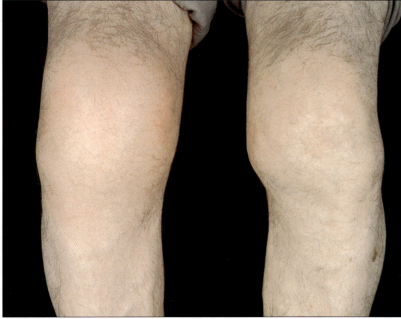

2.3 Acute pseudogout of the right knee. Note swelling and a degree of erythema.

Muscle wasting may be a prominent feature of osteoarthritis. Although general immobility may produce generalized wasting, the most marked wasting is seen in the muscles that act across the affected joint. Location will determine whether this is readily appreciated with some joint involvement: the hip and hand, for example, less likely to produce obvious atrophy than others, such as the knee and shoulder (**2.4**). Although atrophy may be hard to appreciate, the consequence of this may be more easily observed in terms of reduced strength and function. Associated proprioceptive impairment can also result in functional impairment with, for example, impaired gait and balance.

Ligamentous involvement and joint space loss may result in instability and further functional impairment which may manifest as a lack of confidence, falling, and fear of falling. Associated meniscal damage and intra-articular 'loose-bodies' may result in symptoms of 'locking', especially at the knee and elbow (**2.5**) and of 'giving way' (mainly at the knee). Locking is a temporary, painful inability to move the joint in one plane, usually extension, and this often lasts a

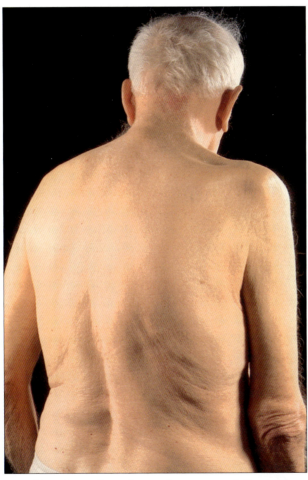

2.4 Global wasting of muscles – especially visible for deltoid, supraspinatus, infraspinatus, and teres minor – in association with right glenohumeral osteoarthritis.

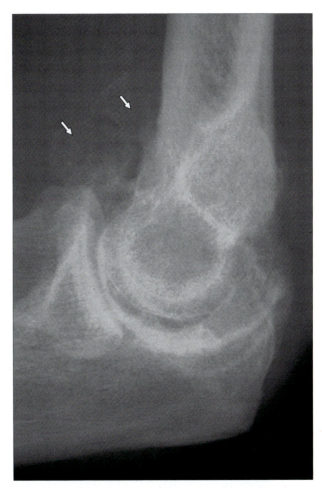

2.5 Osteoarthritis of the elbow showing large osteochondral bodies (arrows). This patient had recurrent locking that required surgical exploration. It was probably the smaller osteochondral bodies, not apparent on this radiograph, that were causing the problem.

34 General features of osteoarthritis

matter of minutes. It is a mechanical problem that results from an interpolation of tissue between the articular surfaces and, if recurrent, may require surgical removal.

'Giving way' is a more difficult concept and has been considered variously as a feeling of instability and lack of confidence in a limb, usually the leg, to a more transient, sudden weakness in the muscles causing a partial but not complete loss of ability to weight-bear, lasting for just a fraction of a second.

Systemic upset is not a feature of osteoarthritis since it is a non-inflammatory condition that does not trigger the acute phase response. An exception is those patients who experience associated calcium crystal synovitis. In this situation, the marked release of inflammatory mediators may result not only in local pain and inflammation, but also fever, myalgia, sweating, and confusion.

What are the radiological features of osteoarthritis?

Joint space narrowing can be appreciated by looking at the intercortical distance between bone separated by hyaline cartilage. The situation is more complex in those joints that contain a fibrocartilage meniscus, such as the tibiofemoral joints of the knee. In this situation, meniscal damage, or indeed surgical removal, will result in a reduced joint space without this necessarily reflecting hyaline cartilage loss. Conversely, at certain sites, such as the knee, a normal joint space width does not exclude significant cartilage loss. This can arise if a non-weight-bearing view is taken (**2.6**) or if the knee is fully extended – a semi-flexed weight-bearing view is optimal and more sensitive at detecting focal cartilage loss. Similarly, the alignment of the x-ray beam relative to the joint may also make a major difference to the appreciation of joint space loss (**2.7**).

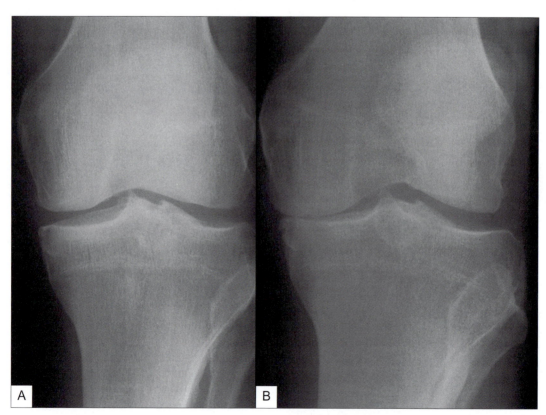

2.6 A non-weight bearing view (**A**) and a weight-bearing view (**B**) of the same knee. The weight-bearing view shows marked medial joint space narrowing that is not apparent on the non-weight bearing view.

The early stages of osteophyte formation involve chondral metaplasia and growth at the joint margins. These early cartilaginous osteophytes are radiolucent and will not be apparent on a plain radiograph. Pathologically, they may be exuberant and, indeed, other imaging modalities (such as MRI) may demonstrate them. These osteophytes tend to develop at the site of capsular and ligamentous insertions. Subsequent ossification occurs and, of course, the associated calcification will cause them to become radio-opaque. In nearly all cases, radiographs will underestimate the size of osteophytes.

Bone growth may occur in other locations. Subchondral bone may demonstrate sclerosis and the trabecular architecture may alter in response to load bearing. This can occur internally leading to thickened trabeculae aligned parallel to stressing forces and externally leading to cortical thickening and periosteal osteophyte or 'buttressing'. The best examples of this are usually seen at the hip (**2.8**).

Bone loss may also be a feature. Typically, this involves subchondral bone leading to altered contour, collapse, and reduced bone height, often as a late feature in association with marked cartilage loss (**2.9**). As previously discussed, localized areas of osteonecrosis may play a role in this. The subchondral loss may also be associated with cyst formation (**2.10**). Prominent multiple cyst formation is more common in patients with haemochromatosis and pyrophosphate arthropathy.

Major focal loss can occur resulting in massive alterations in the cortical outline of a joint. This is most commonly seen at the knee and hip with marked attrition and loss of normal bone outlines (**2.11**).

Finally, appropriate views can identify ossified loose bodies. These are not, as the name implies, floating free within the joint, but are usually embedded in the synovium. They may arise from synoviocytes that undergo metaplasia to cartilage that then ossifies, in which case they may be multiple (**2.12**). Alternatively, they may result from a broken-off fragment of articular cartilage that is then taken up by the synovium and grows and ossifies there, in which case, they may be single or less numerous.

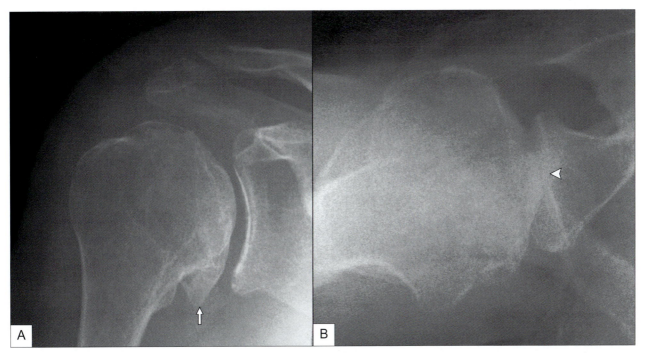

2.7 (**A**) An anteroposterior radiograph of a shoulder which, although showing definite osteophytosis (arrow), appears to demonstrate relatively preserved joint space. On the axial view (**B**) the marked loss of joint space and, by implication, cartilage is readily apparent (arrowhead).

36 General features of osteoarthritis

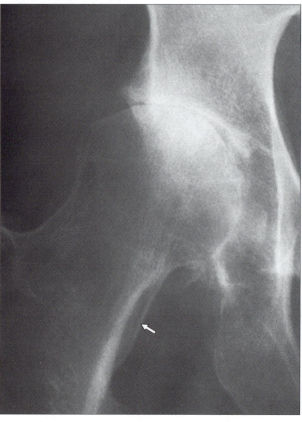

2.8 Radiograph showing marked superior pole hip osteoarthritis with periosteal osteophyte ('buttressing') of the inferior aspect of the femoral neck (arrow).

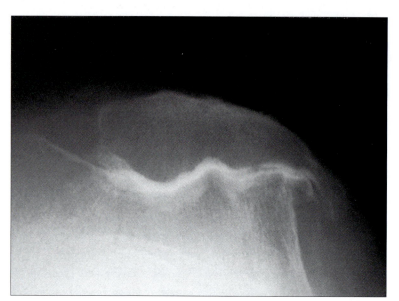

2.9 Skyline view of the patellofemoral joint showing marked cartilage loss of the lateral facet with lateral patella subluxation, sclerosis of subchondral bone, a 'saw-tooth' deformity (ridging of both sides of the joint), and reduced height of the patella.

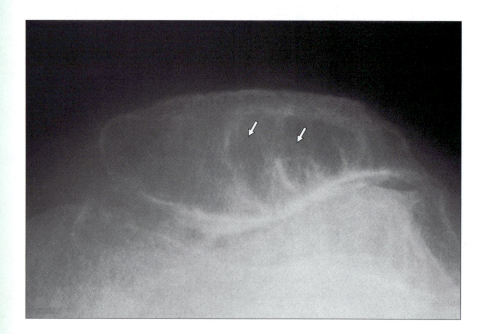

2.10 Skyline view of the patellofemoral compartment showing marked cartilage loss and large well-corticated cysts in the patella (arrows).

2.11 Hip radiograph showing severe superior pole osteoarthritis with complete loss of joint space ('bone-on-bone'), sclerosis, cysts (arrows), and marked loss of bone in the femoral head and acetabulum (arrowhead).

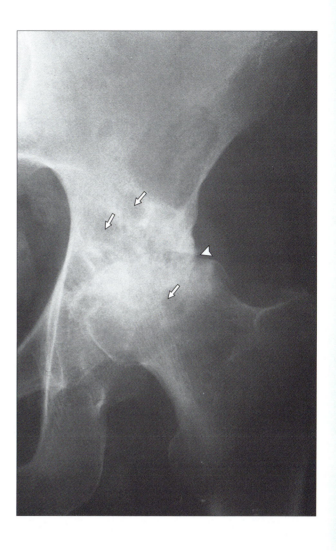

2.12 Hip radiograph showing superior pole osteoarthritis with multiple osteochondral 'loose bodies' (arrows).

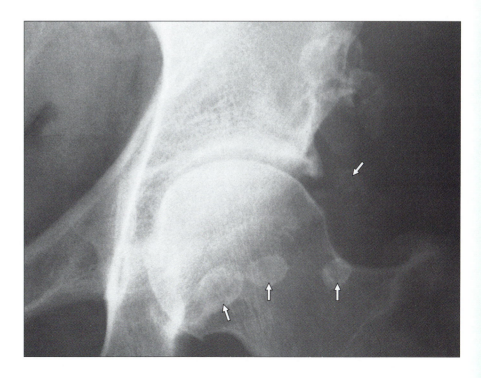

What do other imaging techniques demonstrate in osteoarthritis?

Other imaging techniques can demonstrate the facets of osteoarthritis seen in radiographs to greater or lesser extents. MRI is more sensitive than radiographs in demonstrating cartilage loss, and can also delineate changes in fibro-cartilaginous menisci, synovium, bone, and periarticular structures that are completely invisible on a plain radiograph (**2.13**).

Bone marrow 'oedema' or 'bruising' on MRI, both at the knee (**2.13**) and spine (where it is called Modic change), is more likely to be found in a patient with symptoms, and may predict future progression (**2.14**). The precise pathological nature of this abnormal MRI signal is unclear, but it has been described in vertebral bodies, facet joints, femur, and tibia, and at all these sites a relationship with pain has been described. Other features appreciated on MRI scanning include ligamentous and capsular/synovial change – again not visible on plain radiographs. Cartilage can also be directly measured and quantified and, indeed, measured cartilage volume can be used as a surrogate for joint space narrowing.

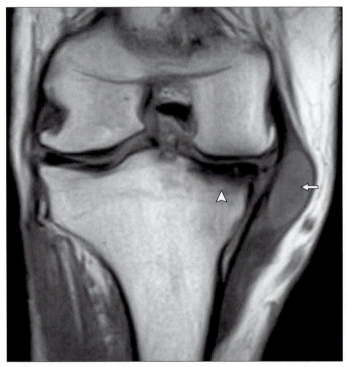

2.13 MRI of an osteoarthritic knee showing osteophyte and cartilage thinning in the medial compartment, but also 'bone oedema' of the upper medial tibia (arrowhead) and medially a very large anserine bursa (arrow) (the source of much of this patient's current pain) – features that are not seen on plain radiographs.

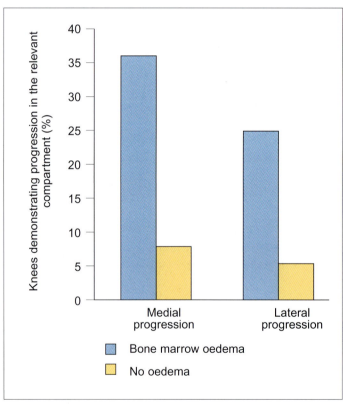

2.14 Relationship of bone marrow oedema to subsequent radiographic progression. (Data derived from Felson DT, McLaughlin S, Goggins J, et al. [2003]. Bone marrow edema and its relation to progression of knee osteoarthritis. *Ann Int Med*, **139**:330–336.)

Ultrasound scanning equipment is generally cheaper than MRI, and newer high-resolution scanners can be used to assess cartilage, osteophytes, and ligaments. In general, however, this is predominantly a research tool at present and is not widely used clinically to assess osteoarthritis.

Radioisotope scanning involves injecting radio-labelled technetium into the circulation and measuring subsequent radioactive emission, both with time and by site. By scanning at appropriate times, this can be used to examine vascularity and perfusion, tissue uptake, and new bone formation. Although not widely used to assess osteoarthritis, it is apparent that bone scan changes related to osteoarthritis are commonly detected in scans performed for other reasons. This requires careful evaluation and differentiation from osteoblastic metastases, inflammatory synovitis, or infection.

At the knee and the hand, radioisotope scanning has been suggested to predict those patients with osteoarthritis who are likely to demonstrate radiographic progression. The predictive value is not high, but certainly patients with 'hotter scans' and with certain scan patterns (such as 'diffuse subchondral bone change' at the knee) (**2.15, 2.16**) are more likely to demonstrate future progression. The clinical usefulness of this finding is not yet clear.

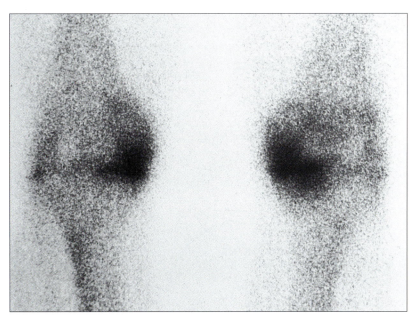

2.15 Radioisotope bone scan (delayed phase) of a patient with knee osteoarthritis showing bilateral diffuse increased uptake in subchondral bone either side of the medial joint lines. This is a pattern that is a risk factor for progressive structural change.

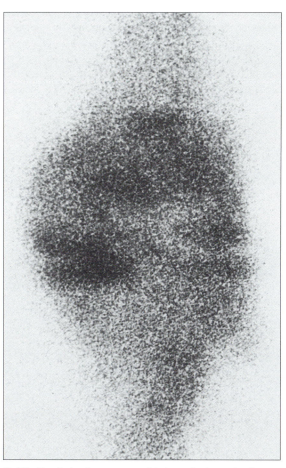

2.16 Radioisotope scan (delayed phase) of an osteoarthritic knee showing a 'tramline' pattern of focal uptake in subchondral bone either side of the medial joint line. This pattern is less likely to progress than that in **2.15**.

Are there subsets of osteoarthritis?

Since the 1960s, there have been suggestions that osteoarthritis may encompass a number of different conditions. The first notion was that in some cases a cause could be identified, usually trauma but occasionally other inflammatory arthritides, leading to division into 'primary' and 'secondary' forms of osteoarthritis. However, such division has been challenged as it is suggested that overt trauma is just one factor in a common complex disorder that merely brings forward the onset of osteoarthritis in otherwise genetically and constitutionally predisposed individuals. The best example of this comes from the study of patients who have undergone meniscectomy in early adult life. Those people who subsequently develop hand osteoarthritis in middle life (i.e. those with a generalized predisposition to osteoarthritis) are more likely to develop post-meniscectomy osteoarthritis at the knee and to have higher x-ray scores, suggesting interaction between extrinsic (trauma) and intrinsic (individual) risk factors.

One way to differentiate subsets of osteoarthritis is simply by the joint involved. Over and above this clinical observation, and epidemiological studies then began to describe patients with particular patterns of involvement of osteoarthritis, although whether these are true distinct entities or simply extreme examples of a continuous spectrum remains unclear. More recent studies have confirmed some of these patterns and have even begun to describe differing genetic and biochemical bases for these. These are now described in more detail (**2.17**).

Further reading

Brandt KD, Doherty M, Lohmander LS (2003). *Osteoarthritis*, 2nd edn, Oxford University Press, Oxford.

Moskowitz RW, Howell DS, Altman RD, *et al.* (2001). *Osteoarthritis: Diagnosis and Medical/Surgical Management.* WB Saunders, London.

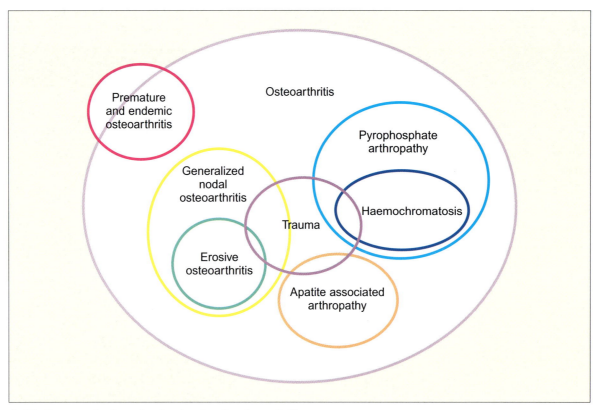

2.17 Commonly described subsets of osteoarthritis.

Chapter 3

Subsets of osteoarthritis

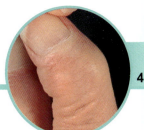

Generalized osteoarthritis

Early epidemiological studies using radiological surveys detailed the fact that many patients had osteoarthritis of multiple joints, suggesting a generalized, in-built predisposition (**3.1**).

Furthermore, the pattern of joint involvement did not appear random, in that certain joints were commonly affected together. In particular, distal interphalangeal joints, medial tibiofemoral compartments, thumb bases, and intervertebral discs and apophyseal joints of the lumbar and cervical spine seemed to be affected quite commonly in the same patients (**3.2**). In addition, many patients were noted to have Heberden's nodes. These occur at the distal interphalangeal joints, and were originally described as 'pea-like swellings' on the posterolateral (radial and ulnar)

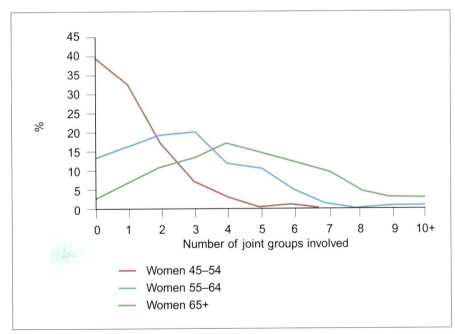
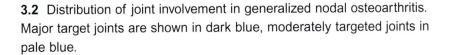
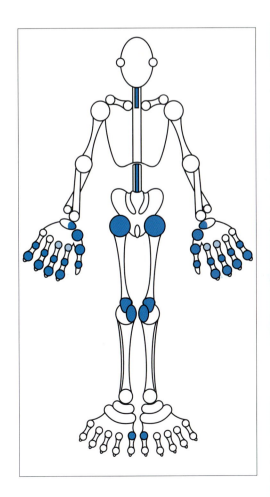

3.1 Accrual of multiple joint involvement with osteoarthritis, and the effect of age.

3.2 Distribution of joint involvement in generalized nodal osteoarthritis. Major target joints are shown in dark blue, moderately targeted joints in pale blue.

aspects of the joint, either side of the extensor tendon. Their early development appears to involve a cystic swelling arising from the synovial cavity of the joint. The cyst contains a gelatinous material which subsequently appears to undergo chondroid metaplasia, and then ossification. Originally, it was unclear if Heberden's nodes always relate to osteoarthritis, but recent studies suggest that the two are closely related. Similar changes can occur at the proximal interphalangeal joints where they are commonly known as Bouchard's nodes (**3.3**).

While multiple Heberden's nodes commonly associate with osteoarthritis at other sites, they may also occur in a few fingers without osteoarthritis elsewhere, perhaps reflecting localized hand trauma. However, multiple nodes commonly associate with polyarticular osteoarthritis in women(**3.4**). The appearance of multiple nodes often occurs around the time of the menopause, and was once known as 'menopausal arthritis'. It is now more commonly termed 'generalized nodal osteoarthritis'. It has a strong genetic component with a marked female preponderance, and a high degree of penetrance, behaving almost like a Mendelian recessive trait.

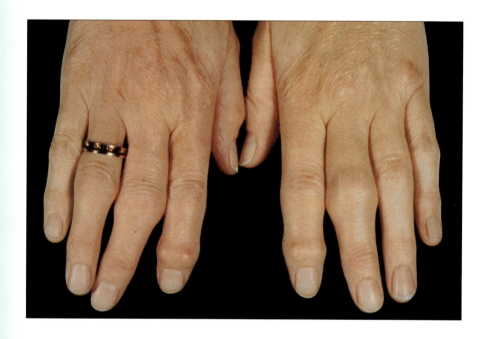

3.3 Nodal osteoarthritis of the hands demonstrating Heberden's nodes at the distal interphalangeal joints, and Bouchard's nodes at the proximal interphalangeal joints. Note additional sideways (radial or ulnar) deviation at some joints – a characteristic deformity of interphalangeal osteoarthritis.

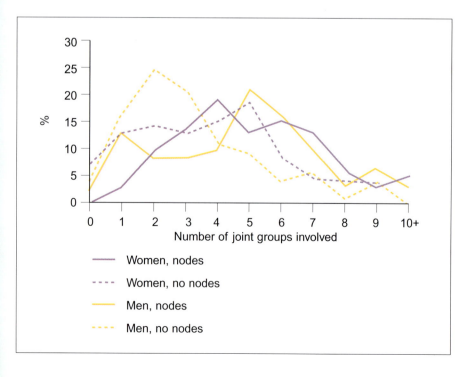

3.4 Numbers of joints involved in both men and women at age >65 years, and the effect of the presence of Heberden's nodes.

Erosive osteoarthritis

Some patients with polyarticular hand osteoarthritis appear to have a worse prognosis. Clinically, this includes a high degree of interphalangeal joint instability (**3.5**), a restricted range of movement, and even joint ankylosis. In addition, there is an almost equal involvement of proximal and distal interphalangeal joints, compared to generalized nodal osteoarthritis where the involvement is predominantly distal.

Radiographically, erosive osteoarthritis is characterized by subchondral erosion of bone. This can give rise to a characteristic 'sea-gull wing' appearance (**3.6**). Bone loss can be marked and lead to finger shortening and, hence, joint laxity. In some cases, there can be late bony fusion (**3.7**). Instability and bony ankylosis are not features of common nodal osteoarthritis.

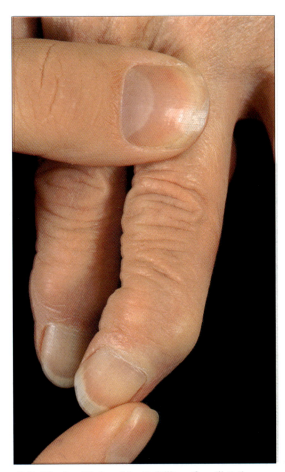

3.5 Marked lateral instability of a distal interphalangeal joint in a patient with 'erosive' osteoarthritis. Such instability is not a feature of common nodal osteoarthritis.

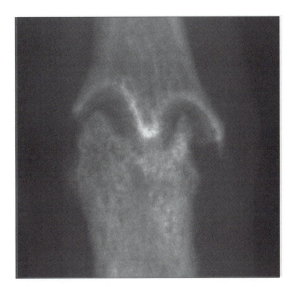

3.6 Erosive osteoarthritis. Marked subchondral erosion leads to scalloping of the bone ends and a 'gull's wing' appearance.

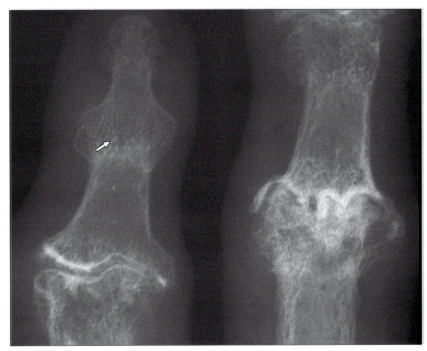

3.7 Erosive osteoarthritis with bony fusion (arrow) of a distal interphalangeal joint.

44 Subsets of osteoarthritis

Pyrophosphate arthropathy

After the nature of gout as a crystal-based arthropathy was elucidated, a group of patients were described in the 1960s with acute self-limiting synovitis of the knee, which clinically resembled gout. However, examination of their aspirated synovial fluid under polarizing light did not reveal the bright, negatively birefringent, needle-shaped crystals of monosodium urate (the gout culprit), but other much smaller, positively birefringent, rhomboid crystals that were chemically identified as calcium pyrophosphate dihydrate (CPPD) crystals (3.8, 3.9). The attacks of acute self-limiting inflammation caused by CPPD crystals were called 'pseudogout'.

Plain radiographs of some patients can also demonstrate calcification of cartilage (chondrocalcinosis) affecting fibro-cartilage and less commonly hyaline cartilage (3.10). Cadaveric and synovial fluid studies have confirmed that usual cause of chondrocalcinosis is CPPD crystal deposition, with other less common causes being apatite and other basic calcium phosphate crystals. Chondrocalcinosis is a common, age-associated radiographic finding that can occur in structurally normal joints. However, there is an increased prevalence of chondrocalcinosis and CPPD crystal deposition in osteoarthritic joints, especially knees, and when they co-exist, the term 'chronic pyrophosphate arthropathy' is often used.

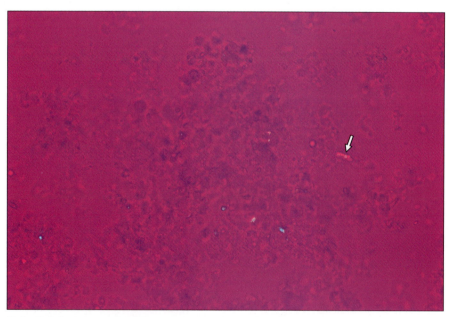

3.8 Calcium pyrophosphate crystals (arrow) in knee synovial fluid (x400 magnification) aspirated during an acute attack of synovitis. The crystals are few in number, small, weakly birefringent, and largely rhomboid in shape.

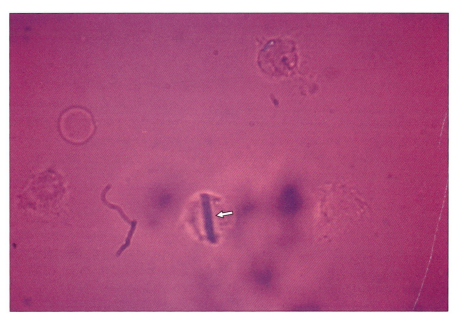

3.9 A higher magnification of the same fluid as in **3.8**, showing an intracellular calcium pyrophosphate crystal that has been phagocytosed by a neutrophil (arrow).

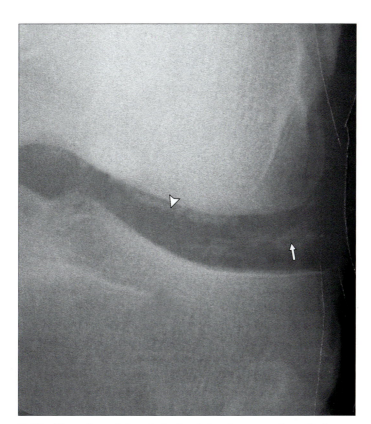

3.10 Chondrocalcinosis in the lateral compartment of a knee. The elongated triangle of calcification in the central, outer half of the joint (arrow) is in the fibrocartilaginous meniscus, whereas the lines of calcification parallel and close to the cortical line (arrowhead) are in hyaline articular cartilage.

While ordinary osteoarthritis and pyrophosphate arthropathy appear very similar, there are some qualitative differences. Apart from the presence of chondrocalcinosis, joints with pyrophosphate arthropathy tend to demonstrate more marked osteophyte, cysts and bone remodelling, resulting in a 'hypertrophic' radiographic appearance (3.11).

The pattern of joint involvement also tends to differ (3.12). In particular, there tends to be more glenohumeral, metacarpophalangeal, midtarsal, and radiocarpal joint involvement – sites that are not commonly targeted for generalized osteoarthritis.

Clinically, apart from possible superimposed acute pseudogout attacks, there is a tendency for more inflammation (stiffness, chronic knee effusions, and soft-tissue swelling) in chronic pyrophosphate arthropathy than uncomplicated osteoarthritis. Chondrocalcinosis and CPPD crystal deposition have also been suggested to be risk factors for more rapid radiographic progression of osteoarthritic structural change at the knee and hip.

Ageing and osteoarthritis are the two common predisposing factors to CPPD crystal deposition and chondrocalcinosis. However, occasionally metabolic diseases that interfere with pyrophosphate metabolism may predispose to chondrocalcinosis (*Table 3.1*) and there are rare kindreds with familial predisposition to florid polyarticular chondrocalcinosis. Such metabolic or familial predisposition should be considered and screened for in patients with polyarticular chondrocalcinosis or if unexplained chondrocalcinosis occurs under age 55. Often there are additional clinical or radiographic clues that suggest metabolic disease (3.13).

Of the metabolic diseases, only haemochromatosis is associated with structural changes resembling osteoarthritis. Haemochromatosis is a disorder of iron storage caused by a

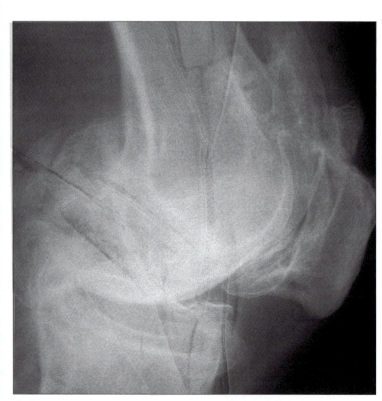

3.11 Lateral knee radiograph of pyrophosphate arthropathy showing a 'hypertrophic' appearance with florid osteophyte formation.

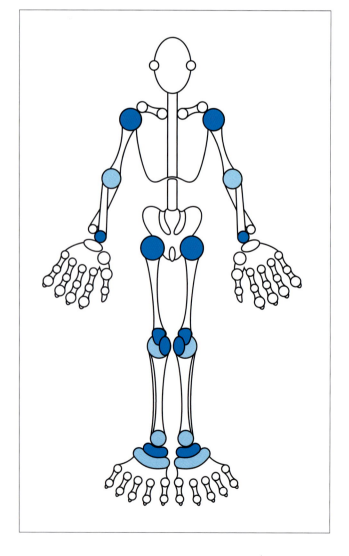

3.12 Distribution of joint involvement in chronic pyrophosphate arthropathy. Major target joints are shown in dark blue, moderately targeted joints in pale blue.

genetic defect in the iron transfer mechanism in the bowel. This results in an accumulation of total body iron with preferential deposition in certain locations, such as endocrine organs, heart, liver, skin, and joints. This can result in diabetes, hypogonadism, hypopituitarism, cardiac failure, liver failure, and diffuse bronzed-skin pigmentation. However, arthritis is very common, and arthropathy can be the presentation of the disease. Haemochromatotic

Table 3.1 Metabolic diseases that predispose to CPPD crystal deposition

Condition	Chondrocalcinosis	Pseudogout	Pyrophosphate arthropathy
Hyperparathyroidism	+	+	–
Haemochromatosis	+	+	+
Hypomagnesaemia	+	+	–
Hypophosphatasia	+	+	–

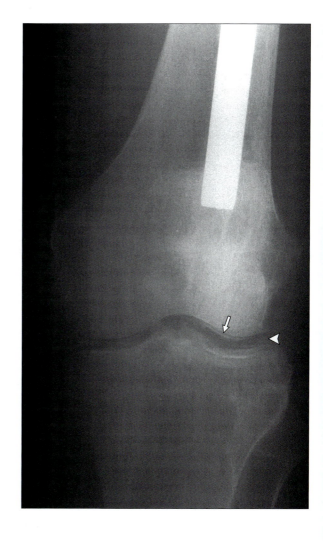

3.13 Knee radiograph of a 50-year-old patient with polyarticular chondrocalcinosis and recurrent pseudogout attacks due to hypophosphatasia. He had also suffered multiple stress fractures, including both femora (hence the surgical rod), from the osteoporosis that results from hypophosphatasia. Note chondrocalcinosis of hyaline cartilage (arrow) and fibrocalcinosis (arrowhead).

48 Subsets of osteoarthritis

arthopathy has many similarities to pyrophosphate arthropathy, but may be suspected particularly if there is involvement of metacarpophalangeal joints, and if multiple subchondral cysts are a prominent feature.

Familial forms of chondrocalcinosis behave as autosomal dominant monogenic disorders, and in some families mutations of the ANKH (ankylosis human) gene that result in excessive extracellular pyrophosphate levels have been identified. Some families develop chondrocalcinosis alone (**3.14, 3.15**), whereas others develop structural changes of pyrophosphate arthropathy.

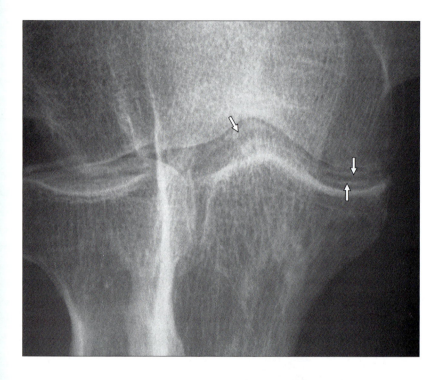

3.14 Elbow radiograph of a 45-year-old patient with familial chondrocalcinosis who had suffered recurrent pseudogout attacks at multiple joint sites. He had florid chondrocalcinosis of many joints (arrows).

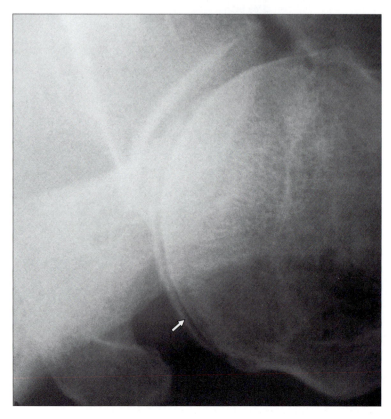

3.15 Shoulder radiograph of the same patient as in **3.14** showing chondrocalcinosis of hyaline cartilage over the humeral head (arrow).

Apatite associated destructive arthritis (AADA)

Apatite and other basic calcium phosphate (BCP) crystals are too small to be seen using conventional light microscopy. However, aggregates of BCP crystals in synovial fluid or synovium can be seen using calcium stains, such as Alizarin red S (**3.16**). The relationship of these crystals to osteoarthritis is not totally clear, but they are commonly found in synovial fluid of osteoarthritic knees and may co-exist with CPPD crystals ('mixed crystal deposition').

Intra-articular apatite and BCP crystals were described initially in association with a rapidly progressive form of osteoarthritis affecting large joints (hips, knees, and shoulders) of elderly people, especially women (**3.17**).

At the shoulder this is commonly known as 'Milwaukee shoulder'. AADA is often very painful and associates, at the knee and shoulder, with large cool effusions and often marked instability. It has a poor prognosis and usually requires joint replacement. The radiographs show 'atrophic' changes with marked bone attrition and very little if any osteophyte (**3.18, 3.19**). At the hip and knee, there may be widening of the joint space, reflecting the marked loss of cartilage and subchondral bone (**3.20**), though stressed, weight-bearing views usually bring the bone ends together. The differential diagnosis is septic arthritis, late osteonecrosis or neuropathic joint.

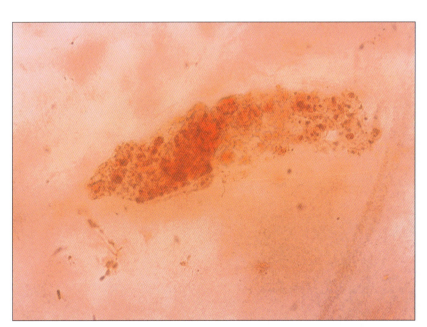

3.16 Alizarin red S stained synovial fluid showing aggregates of basic calcium phosphate crystals.

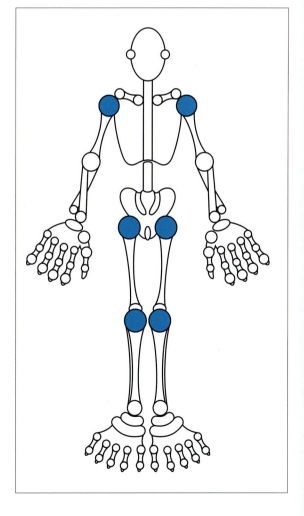

3.17 Target joints affected by AADA.

50 Subsets of osteoarthritis

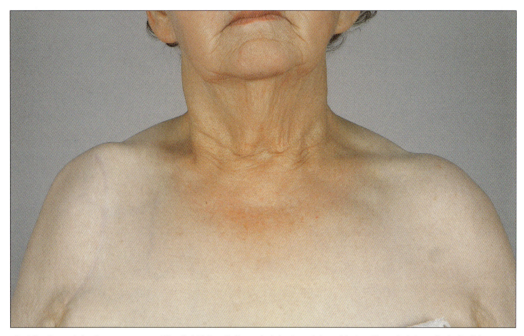

3.18 An elderly woman with AADA of the right shoulder. Note the right subdeltoid swelling due to a large effusion that communicates with the subacromial space and glenohumeral joint.

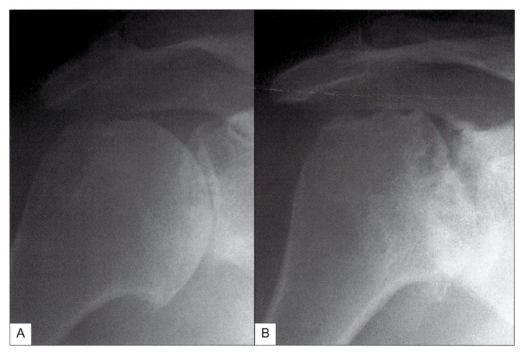

3.19 Shoulder radiographs of the same patient as in **3.18**. The first radiograph (**A**) was obtained at onset of her symptoms and shows narrowing, sclerosis and osteophyte at the glenohumeral joint. The second radiograph (**B**), taken just 4 months later, shows rapid progression with marked bone loss either side of the joint.

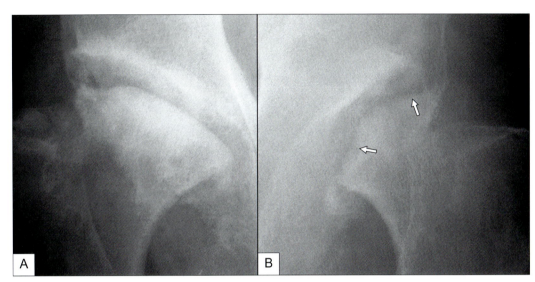

3.20A, B Two examples of AADA of the hip. Both patients came to joint surgery. Note the marked 'atrophic' appearance with marked bone attrition (arrows) and apparent joint space widening.

Premature onset osteoarthritis

Osteoarthritis is principally a condition of the middle-aged and elderly and, in general, is ubiquitous throughout the world. If osteoarthritis occurs at a younger age, or if an atypical distribution is seen, then a search for a predisposing cause should be made (*Table 1.2*, page 20). Since the communities affected by endemic osteoarthritis are often disadvantaged, it is unusual to see subjects with this outside of endemic areas. Nevertheless, the family history may be relevant, and a full general medical enquiry and examination should be undertaken. Radiographs may give additional clues (e.g. dysplasia, chondrocalcinosis) and further targeted tests for metabolic or endocrine disease might be required.

Having excluded known predisposing causes, most causes of 'premature' osteoarthritis are limited to one or a few joints, and are explained by prior trauma or arthropathy. Nevertheless, there remain some patients with apparently sporadic, often symmetrical, osteoarthritis that presents in their 4th decade. It is unclear whether this represents a truly distinctive form of arthritis, or merely represents the 'tail' of the distribution of age of onset.

Further reading

Brandt KD, Doherty M, Lohmander LS (2003). *Osteoarthritis*, 2nd edn, Oxford University Press, Oxford.

Moskowitz RW, Howell DS, Altman RD, *et al.* (2001). *Osteoarthritis: Diagnosis and Medical/Surgical Management.* WB Saunders, London.

Chapter 4

Features of osteoarthritis at specific sites

Features of osteoarthritis of the knee

The knee is comprised of one synovial cavity with three principle compartments: the medial and lateral tibiofemoral joints, and the patellofemoral joint. Any or all of these compartments may be affected by osteoarthritis, although different patterns of involvement occur and may be associated with different epidemiological risk factors.

Since the knee is a large and relatively superficial joint, the signs of osteoarthritis can be easily appreciated clinically. Modest synovitis results in local warmth and joint effusion. Small effusions tend to fill in the sulci on the medial and lateral aspects of patellae. Larger effusions tend to open up the large suprapatellar pouch, presenting a swelling above and to either side of the patella.

There is a natural weak point in the posterior aspect of the knee capsule, and with any synovial effusion there is a potential for a cyst-like protrusion to form known as a 'popliteal' or Baker's cyst (**4.1**). This may cause localized posterior pain, and may expand into the calf as a calf cyst.

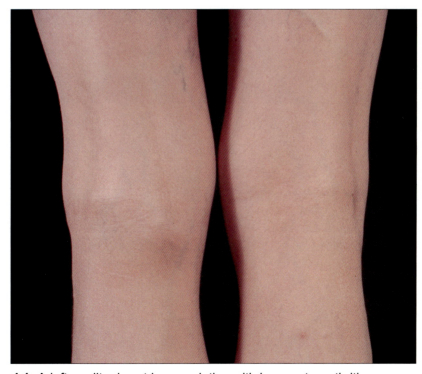

4.1 A left popliteal cyst in association with knee osteoarthritis.

Course crepitus is a common feature of osteoarthritis, and is readily appreciated by holding the front of the knee as it moves. It probably reflects fibrillation of the articular cartilage, or eventually bone rubbing on bone, and hence friction on movement. Bony swelling, i.e. osteophyte, can be palpated and often seen, particularly on the medial and lateral aspects of the knee.

Varus (**4.2**) and valgus (**4.3**) deformities should be assessed standing, since they are then maximized. Varus is the more common since osteoarthritis targets the medial more than the lateral tibiofemoral compartment. Fixed flexion deformity is also common. It may be obvious with the patient standing, but mild degrees are best assessed with the patient lying down and pushing both knees backwards onto the couch. This manoeuvre also allows detection of quadriceps wasting, which is common and often exaggerated by the extent of the bony swelling.

The pattern of compartmental involvement has, for many

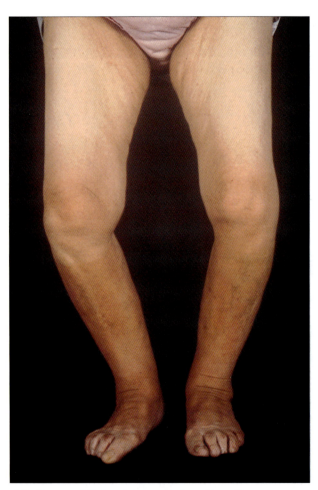

4.2 Severe bilateral varus deformity, with accompanying fixed flexion, in an elderly woman with knee osteoarthritis.

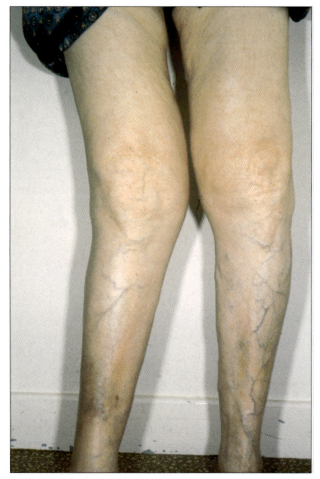

4.3 Gross right valgus and mild left varus deformity in a patient with osteoarthritis. This asymmetrical combination is sometimes called 'windswept' or 'skier's' knees.

years, been masked by the limited extent to which structural involvement was determined by radiology. Many early studies employed only a single anteroposterior, non-weight-bearing view which often underestimates the degree of tibiofemoral involvement and completely ignores the patellofemoral joint. It is now recognized that loading the tibiofemoral compartment, by taking the radiograph with the patient standing, allows a better estimate of the inter-cortical distance. Furthermore, a semi-flexed position brings the maximally affected cartilage into the weight-bearing position and increases the sensitivity of detecting tibio-femoral narrowing. It is now recognized that the patello-femoral compartment is commonly affected by osteoarthritis and indeed is a common cause of anterior knee pain. Osteophyte can be readily recognized using most standard radiographic techniques, but joint space narrowing is best appreciated using an axial view (**4.4**).

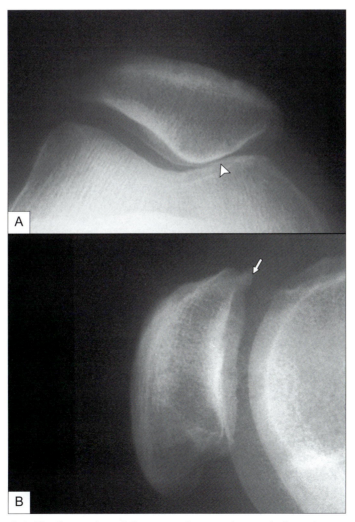

4.4 Radiographs of the same knee using a skyline view (**A**) and lateral flexion view (**B**). On the skyline view, there is marked narrowing of the medial aspect of the patellofemoral joint (arrowhead) that is not apparent on the lateral view. The lateral view, however, demonstrates superior patellar osteophyte (arrow) though no osteophyte is seen on the skyline view.

Using sensitive imaging techniques, it is apparent that most cases of knee osteoarthritis involve all three compartments to some extent, but cartilage narrowing usually predominates in just one or two compartments. Osteophytes are often more widespread at many sites within the knee, and tend to show characteristic directions of growth. For example, in the medial tibiofemoral compartment, they tend to grow horizontally and then away from the joint line (**4.5**); whereas in the lateral tibiofemoral compartment, the femoral osteophyte grows proximally away from the joint line, but the tibial osteophyte often grows vertically towards the femur (**4.6**). In the patellofemoral compartment, lateral subluxation is common (readily seen on the skyline view) and osteophyte tends to grow laterally, hugging the femoral contour (**4.7**). Lateral views show osteophyte superiorly and inferiorly, and often enthesophyte at the quadriceps and patella tendon insertion sites (**4.8**). Presumably, these differences in osteophyte direction are driven by biomechanical forces. Surgical removal of tibiofemoral osteophytes has been shown to increase joint movement, so the osteophytes appear to be a stabilizing factor that help splint the osteoarthritic joint as it loses cartilage and remodels its shape.

Osteochondral bodies are not infrequent within the capsule and ligaments of the joints (**4.9**), and may relate to locking, if close to the joint line. Chondrocalcinosis is readily appreciated in the knee, and 80% of cases of chondrocalcinosis are apparent on anteroposterior radiographs. Calcification occurs in the fibro- and hyaline cartilage and may also be apparent in the capsule of the joint (**4.10**).

Predominant medial tibiofemoral osteoarthritis appears to be particularly common in men. Associated meniscal degeneration is usually a feature, and is more often appreciated if other imaging modalities (such as MRI) are used. Varus deformity, often with fixed flexion if severe, is the most common deformity in men with knee osteoarthritis. Varus deformity is a risk factor for more rapid X-ray progression.

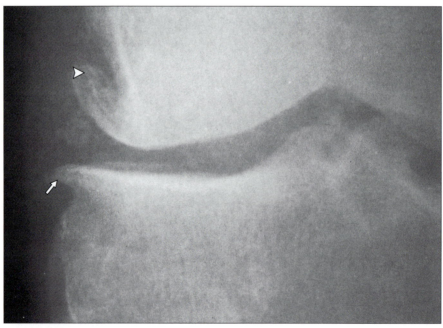

4.5 Medial tibiofemoral osteophytes, growing horizontally (arrow) or away (arrowhead) from each other.

Features of osteoarthritis at specific sites

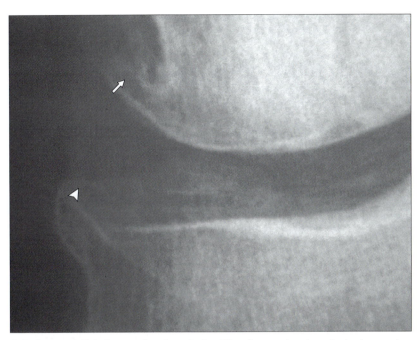

4.6 Lateral tibiofemoral osteophyte. The femoral osteophyte (arrow) is growing proximally away from the joint, but the tibial osteophye (arrowhead) can be seen coming upwards towards the joint.

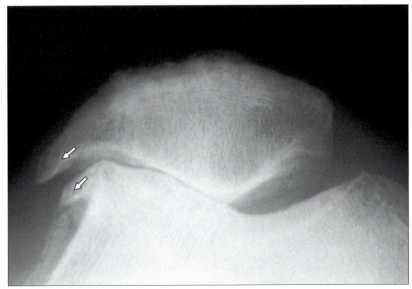

4.7 Skyline view showing marked lateral narrowing, lateral patella subluxation, and osteophytes on both the femoral and patella aspects (arrows), following a similar direction of growth.

58 Features of osteoarthritis at specific sites

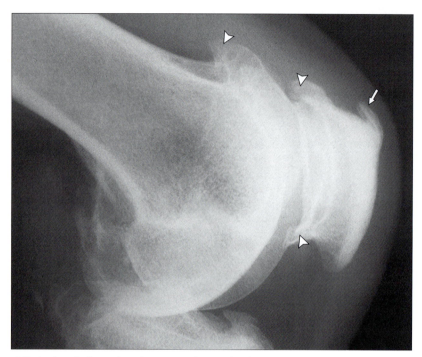

4.8 Lateral view showing superior and inferior patellar and femoral osteophytes (arrowheads), and enthesophyte (arrow) at the quadriceps tendon insertion into the anterior/superior aspect of the patella.

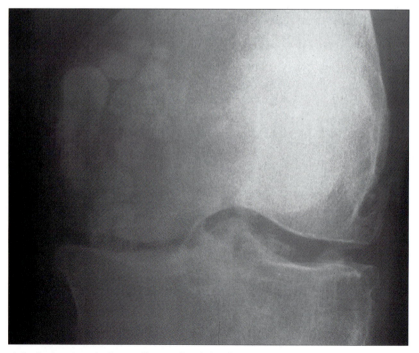

4.9 Anteroposterior radiograph of the knee demonstrating marked osteochondral body formation.

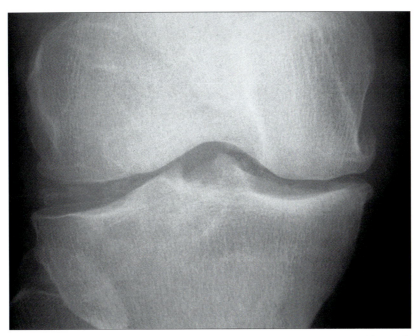

4.10 Knee radiograph showing medial tibiofemoral osteoarthritis and chondrocalcinosis of fibrocartilage and hyaline cartilage ('pyrophosphate arthropathy').

Predominant patellofemoral osteoarthritis is also common, particularly in women. Since the patella is intimately involved in the quadriceps mechanism, muscle wasting and disability appear to be a prominent feature of patellofemoral osteoarthritis. Characteristics of patellofemoral pain include well-localized anterior knee pain, particularly bad when going up or down stairs or an incline, and progressive aching anteriorly when sitting, relieved by getting up and 'stretching the legs.'

The third most common pattern is a combination of both patellofemoral and medial tibiofemoral osteoarthritis. The more knee compartments involved, and the more severe the structural changes, the more likely it is to detect calcium pyrophosphate or apatite crystals in aspirated knee synovial fluid.

Isolated lateral tibiofemoral osteoarthritis is a very uncommon pattern. However, pathological involvement is often present, and it may be that the natural varus deformity (common in medial tibiofemoral osteoarthritis) tends to open up the lateral tibiofemoral joint. If this is the case, cartilage loss in this compartment is not readily appreciated radiographically. Predominant involvement of the lateral tibiofemoral joint may be associated with preceding trauma, previous lateral meniscectomy, or apatite-associated destructive arthritis (**4.11**). A valgus deformity is the usual consequence of severe involvement.

In contrast to osteoarthritis, chronic inflammatory synovitis, such as occurs with rheumatoid arthritis, usually results in a diffuse tricompartmental pattern of joint space loss and little, if any, bone response (**4.12**).

The superior tibiofibular joint is the final joint of the knee. Although radiographic osteoarthritis and often marked cystic change (**4.13**) can occur at this joint, it is rarely a cause of symptoms. Cystic change at this site is more common in patients with knee chondrocalcinosis.

60 Features of osteoarthritis at specific sites

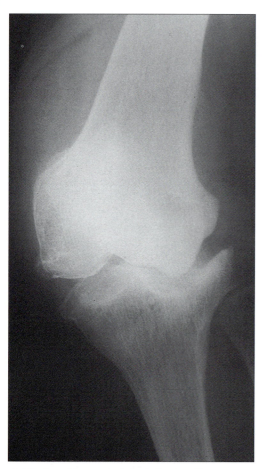

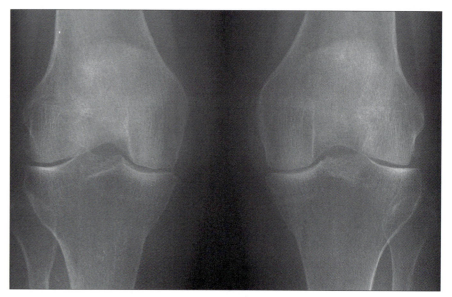

4.12 Knee radiographs of a patient with rheumatoid arthritis showing diffuse joint space narrowing with osteopenia, and without osteophyte or sclerosis.

4.11 Apatite-associated destructive arthritis targeting the lateral tibiofemoral compartment of an elderly woman. Note the severe bone attrition, valgus deformity, and soft-tissue outline of a large effusion.

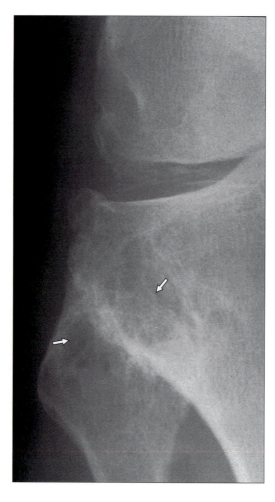

4.13 Marked cystic change (arrows) each side of the superior tibiofibular joint in a patient with pyrophosphate arthropathy of the knee.

Features of osteoarthritis of the hip

Osteoarthritis of the hip is a common clinical problem, and is responsible for a great deal of pain and suffering, as well as being the main indication for hip arthroplasty. Unlike osteoarthritis elsewhere, it shows an overall equal sex distribution, but it predominates in younger men (pre-retirement age) and in elderly women. The principle clinical feature is pain. This is usually felt anteriorly, deep in the groin. It may, however, radiate widely and can be felt in the anteromedial thigh, buttock or the anteromedial aspect of the knee, and may extend as far as the ankle. It can present as knee pain alone, and this may lead to clinical confusion until the knee and hip are both examined.

Restriction of movement commonly occurs and may be relatively painless. The restriction initially affects internal rotation of the hip, particularly in flexion (**4.14**). Later a flexion deformity of the hip occurs, and the patient may walk with a flexed knee to compensate and a degree of equinus. Leg length shortening, due to both the flexion deformity and possibly loss of joint space, can result in a compensatory scoliosis. At an even later stage, a fixed adduction and external rotation of the hip can occur (**4.15, 4.16**).

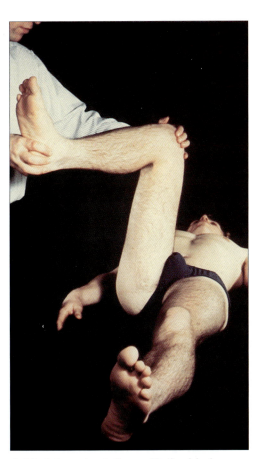

4.14 Internal rotation with the hip in flexion. This is first movement to become painful and restricted with hip arthropathy, and is the most sensitive clinical test for early hip osteoarthritis.

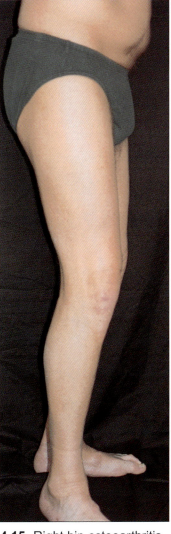

4.15 Right hip osteoarthritis in a 59-year-old man, showing the typical deformity of hip flexion (with compensatory knee flexion) and external rotation.

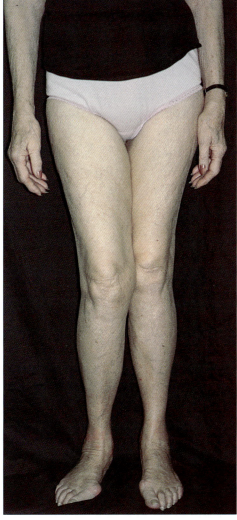

4.16 Advanced right hip osteoarthritis in an elderly woman, showing typical late deformity of hip (and knee) flexion, external rotation, and adduction at the hip.

Muscle wasting is not readily appreciated at the hip, especially in elderly patients, although gluteal and quadriceps wasting is often present. Acute synovitis can occur, including pseudogout, but appears to be unusual in clinical practice. Functional limitation is often a major problem through interference with daily activities, such as putting on socks, getting in and out of cars, and walking.

Radiographically, osteoarthritis of the hip tends to be a focal disease with regard to joint space loss. Superior-narrowing is the most common pattern, especially in men, though focal-narrowing may also be axial or medial (**4.17**). The superior pattern may be predominantly superolateral (**4.18**), and associate eventually with upwards and outwards subluxation of the femoral head, or superomedial. The medial (**4.19**) or axial patterns are less common (**4.20**), but an axial pattern, in particular, may result in a *protrusio acetabulae* abnormality (**4.21**).

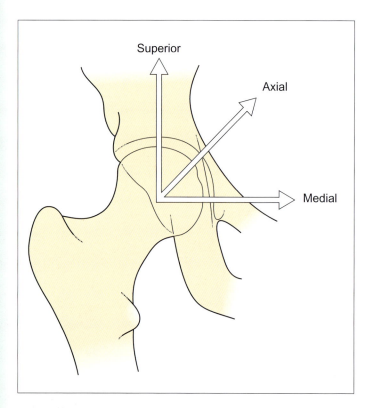

4.17 Diagram showing the different sites for focal narrowing at the hip.

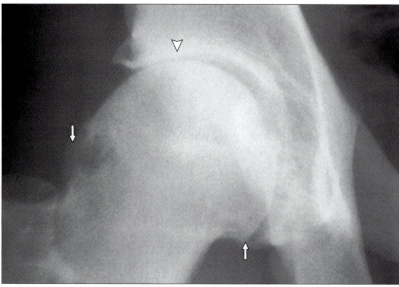

4.18 Superolateral narrowing in hip osteoarthritis. There is also osteophyte on the femoral head (arrows), and sclerosis at the site of maximal narrowing (arrowhead).

Features of osteoarthritis at specific sites

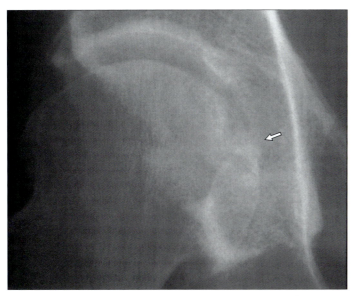

4.19 Medial narrowing in hip osteoarthritis (arrow).

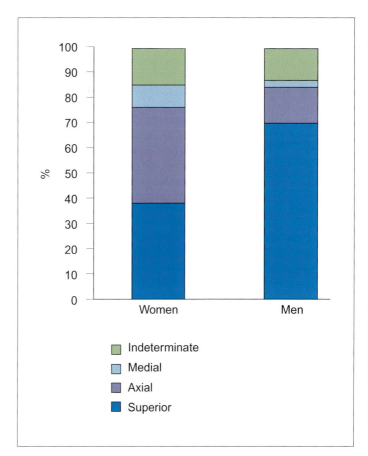

4.20 Different patterns of osteoarthritis of the hip. (Data derived from a sibling study of hip osteoarthritis by Lanyon P, Muir K, Doherty S, et al. [2004]. Influence of radiographic phenotype on risk of hip osteoarthritis within families. *ARD*, **63**:259–263.)

4.21 *Protrusio acetabulae* abnormality – the femoral head has migrated axially, narrowing the acetabular bone and pushing it inwards into the pelvis (arrowheads).

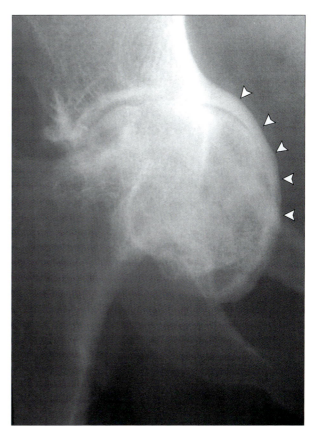

64 Features of osteoarthritis at specific sites

Sometimes, especially with late, marked osteoarthritis, a discrete pattern is hard to discern (an 'indeterminate' pattern). A uniform concentric pattern of cartilage loss is very rare and, especially if there is paucity of accompanying osteophyte, should always suggest an underlying inflammatory or metabolic disease.

Unless there is a specific localizing factor in operation, such as prior trauma, the pattern of involvement is usually identical if osteoarthritis affects both hips.

Osteophyte occurs at specific locations which can include the acetabular margin, and the site of capsular insertion on the femur where it may appear as a line across the femoral head, which is in reality a two-dimensional view of a ring of osteophyte (**4.22**). Cortical buttressing may occur, as well as trabecular thickening. The latter tends to occur parallel to the forces acting on the femoral neck, and thus buttress the medial aspect of the femoral neck. Chondrocalcinosis may be seen occasionally in the hyaline cartilage of the femur (**4.23**), and in the acetabular labrum, though it is more prevalent in the symphysis pubis (**4.24**). Osteochondral bodies may be seen around the joint, with some appearing to form as extensions to acetabular osteophyte.

Cyst formation can occur in the acetabulum, and is particularly common in patients with pyrophosphate arthropathy, especially in association with haemochromatosis (**4.25**). Avascular necrosis of the femoral head can sometimes be appreciated as a focal-marked loss of bone stock.

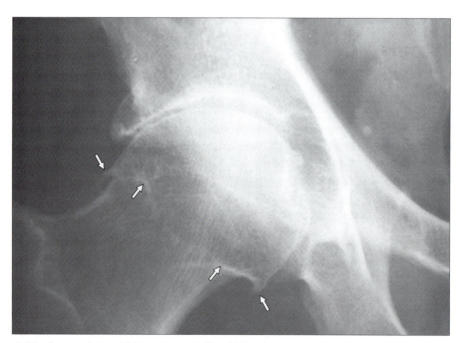

4.22 Superolateral hip osteoarthritis. Note the osteophyte (arrows) that is forming a collar around the margins of the femoral head, appearing as a wavy line crossing the femoral neck in this two-dimensional radiograph.

4.23 Hip chondrocalcinosis affecting the femoral head hyaline cartilage, just visible superolaterally (arrow).

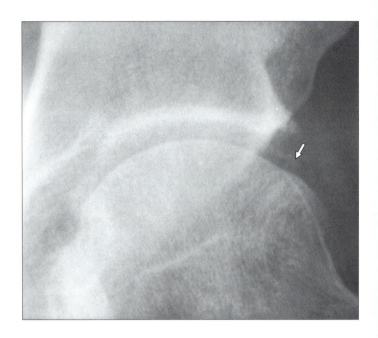

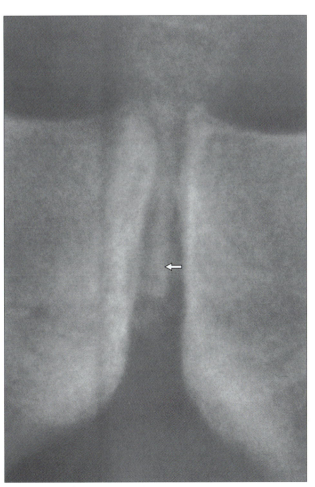

4.24 Chondrocalcinosis (arrow) of the symphysis pubis (the most common site for chondrocalcinosis in the pelvis).

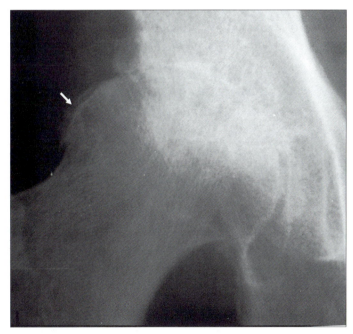

4.25 Hip radiograph in a patient with haemochromatosis. Note the diffuse narrowing and multiple small cysts. An additional clue to underlying metabolic disease is chondrocalcinosis of hyaline cartilage, seen laterally on the femoral head (arrow).

66 Features of osteoarthritis at specific sites

There has been discussion as to how much dysplasia might predispose to osteoarthritis. It appears to be an unusual cause of sporadic osteoarthritis, but occasionally patients presenting with osteoarthritis show clear evidence of acetabular dysplasia, or even possible congenital dislocation of the hip. Prior trauma leading to leg length shortening or malalignment may be appreciated. All these factors have been implicated in determining speed of progression in hip osteoarthritis, but recent meta-analyses suggest that only some of these may be important (*Table 4.1*).

Paget's disease is common in the pelvis, and may affect the acetabulum with resultant hip osteoarthritis, often with diffuse joint space narrowing (**4.26**).

Table 4.1 Hip osteoarthritis: factors associated with progression

Good evidence for a positive effect
- Superolateral migration of the femoral head
- Atrophic bone response

Good evidence for no effect
- Body mass index
- Hip dysplasia

Lievense AM, Bierma-Zeinstra SMA, Verhagen AP, et al. (2002). Prognostic factors of progress of hip osteoarthritis: a systematic review. *Arthritis Care Res*, 47:556–562.

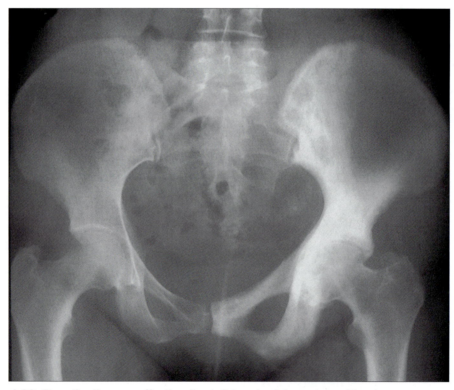

4.26 Paget's disease affecting the left hemipelvis and resulting in osteoarthritis. Note the diffuse, rather than focal narrowing at the hip.

Features of osteoarthritis of the hand and wrist

All joints of the hand and wrist can potentially be affected by osteoarthritis (**4.27, 4.28**), although certain patterns of involvement are characteristic. Distal interphalangeal joint involvement is particularly common, often as part of generalized nodal osteoarthritis. Clinically, this usually starts with development of painful Heberden's nodes around the time of the menopause. These often appear cystic or soft in the early stages of development (**4.29**) and occur at the superolateral aspects of the joint. Once established, the two superolateral swellings either side of the extensor tendon may fuse to form a hard bony posterior bar (**4.30**). Nail dystrophy with ridging ('Heberden's nodes nails') is an occasional associated feature (**4.29**). Varying degrees of inflammation can be appreciated while the nodes evolve to their final form. The onset tends to be stuttering with sequential involvement of new joints, often in a symmetrical fashion, with earlier involvement of the dominant hand.

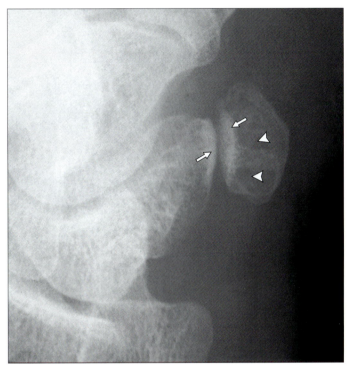

4.27 Osteoarthritis of the pisiform bone of the wrist. Note sclerosis (arrows), cyst formation (arrowheads) and joint space loss.

4.28 Accrual of joint involvement by age and gender in a Finnish population. (Data derived from Haara MM, Kroger H, Arokoski JP, et al. [2003]. Osteoarthritis of finger joints in Finns aged 30 or over. Prevalence, determinants and association with mortality. *ARD*, **62**:151–158.)

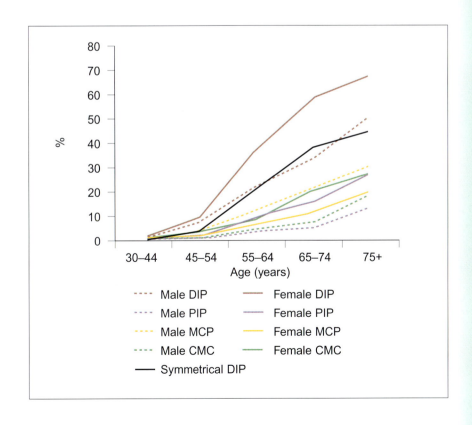

68 Features of osteoarthritis at specific sites

Radiographically, joint space narrowing, sclerosis, osteophytes, and cysts may all occur (**4.31**). Similar involvement of the proximal interphalangeal joints forming Bouchard's nodes may occur, although this is less common. Although usually symptomatic for several years while evolving, Heberden's and Bouchard's nodes often become asymptomatic once fully developed and the prognosis, with respect to subsequent hand function, is usually good.

Gout has a tendency to develop in previously-damaged joints and in post-menopausal women, particularly those on long-term diuretics (thiazides or loop diuretics). Gouty tophi may form at the site of distal interphalangeal osteoarthritis (**4.32**). In severe cases, acute inflammation may occur; and with chronic deposition, the tophi may grow very large, and may even ulcerate and discharge white tophaceous material (**4.33**).

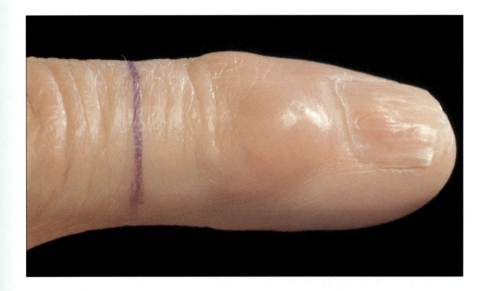

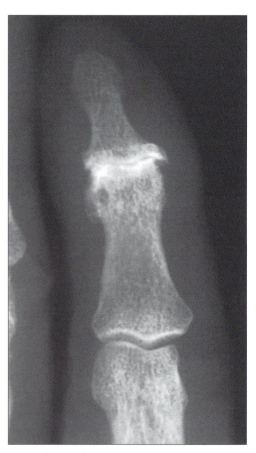

4.29 Superolateral cystic change in an early Heberden's node. Note the accompanying nail dystrophy.

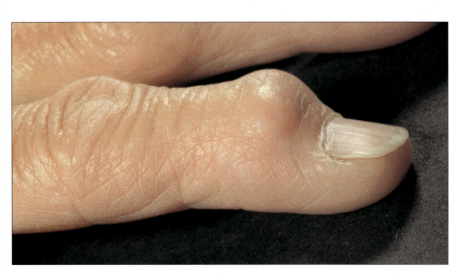

4.30 Established Heberden's node forming a single hard bar over the superior aspect of the joint.

4.31 Radiograph showing distal interphalangeal osteoarthritis in association with a Heberden's node, showing narrowing, osteophyte, sclerosis, and cysts.

Features of osteoarthritis at specific sites

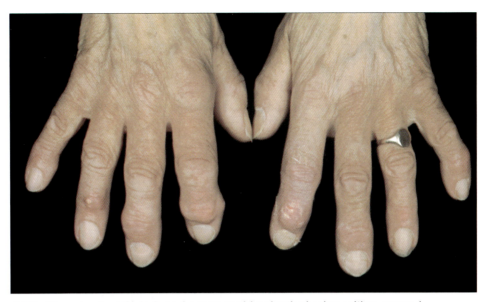

4.32 Chronic diuretic-induced gouty tophi selectively depositing around Heberden's nodes. The white colour of the monosodium urate crystal deposits can easily be seen.

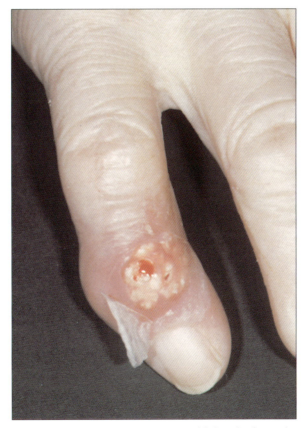

4.33 An ulcerating tophus on a Heberden's node.

Features of osteoarthritis at specific sites

In the variant known as 'erosive osteoarthritis,' the involvement of distal and proximal interphalangeal joints is more equal. Clinically, ligamentous instability seems more common, and lateral and medial deviations of the joint may be seen either at rest or on stressing the joint (**3.5**). In addition, bony fusion may lead to stiffness and rigidity of the joints. Therefore, the functional impairment that results from this form of finger osteoarthritis is often high. Subchondral erosion is the hallmark of this condition, and may give rise to a typical 'gull's wing' appearance, and sometimes resultant bony ankylosis (**3.6, 3.7**).

Involvement of the 'thumb base' is common. Pain from this site is felt mainly in the snuff box area of the radial side of the wrist, although it often radiates proximally into the lateral border of the forearm, and distally up the thumb metacarpal. The pain may be provoked on examination by extending and adducting the thumb, and is often made worse by gripping. Bony swelling and subluxation may

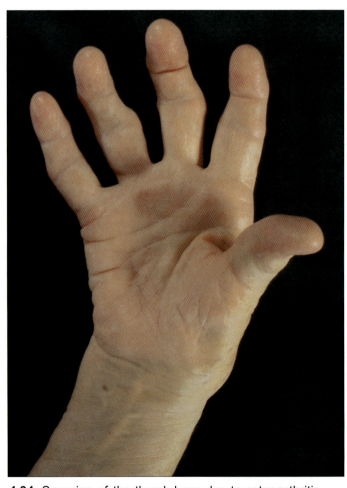

4.34 Squaring of the thumb base due to osteoarthritis. Note the accompanying wasting of the thenar eminence.

Features of osteoarthritis at specific sites

result in squaring of the thumb base, and wasting and weakness of the thenar muscles may occur (**4.34**).

Radiographically there may be involvement of either the scaphotrapezoid or the trapeziometacarpophalangeal joint, or both (**4.35**). Joint space narrowing and sclerosis are often the main features, though osteophyte and cysts may also occur.

Metacarpophalangeal joint involvement, mainly affecting the index and middle finger joints, is relatively uncommon and should lead to consideration of pyrophosphate arthropathy and haemochromatosis. However, it may occur in more elderly patients with nodal generalized osteoarthritis, or in men who have physically demanding occupations ('Missouri arthropathy'). Clinically bony swelling of the joint is seen (**4.36**) together with crepitus and occasional soft-tissue swelling. The appearance can be so marked as to lead to possible confusion with the changes seen in rheumatoid arthritis. Radiographically there may be

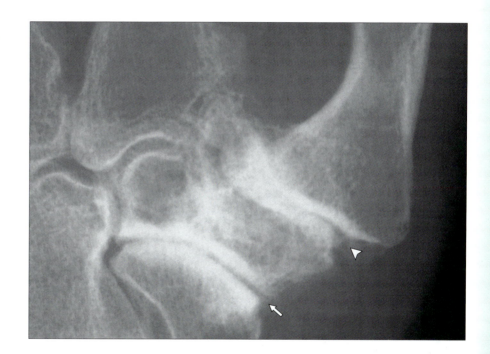

4.35 Radiograph showing osteoarthritis of the scaphotrapezoid (arrow) and trapeziometacarpophalangeal joints (arrowhead) with sclerosis and narrowing the main features.

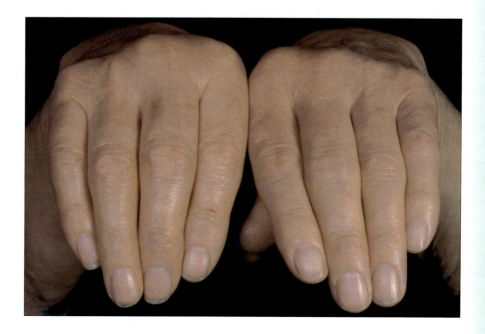

4.36 Prominent bony swelling of the index and middle metacarpophalangeal joints due to osteoarthritis in a 62-year-old man who had a physically demanding job as a machinist.

Features of osteoarthritis at specific sites

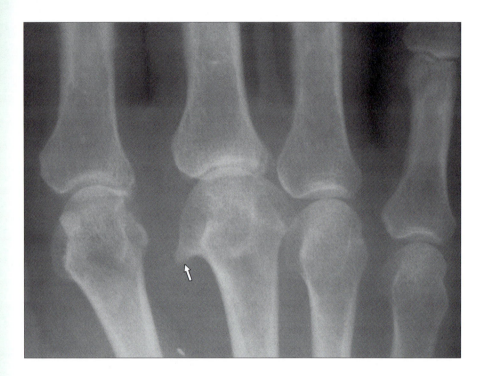

4.37 Hand radiograph of the patient in **4.36**. Note the narrowing of both affected metacarpophalangeal joints and the large 'hook' osteophyte (arrow) on the radial aspect of the middle finger metacarpal head.

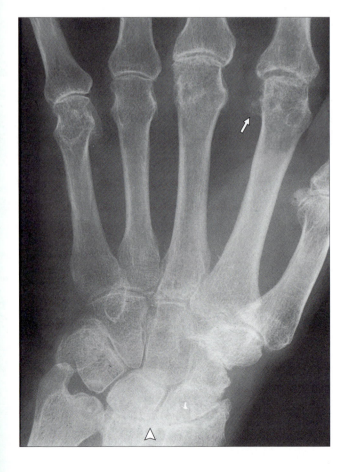

4.38 Haemachromatotic arthropathy. Note involvement of the metacarpophalangeal joints with 'hook' osteophytes on the ulnar border (arrow). Note additional involvement of the radiocarpal joint and multiple small cysts at that site (arrowhead).

joint space narrowing, sclerosis, cysts, and osteophyte. Large 'hook' osteophytes, mainly on the radial side of the distal metacarpal, may be striking (**4.37**). In haemochromatosis there may be more widespread involvement of all metacarpophalangeal joints, additional involvement of the radiocarpal and midcarpal joints, multiple subchondral bone cysts and chondrocalcinosis (**4.38**).

Involvement of the radiocarpal joint is relatively uncommon, but more likely to occur in the context of pyrophosphate arthropathy or previous trauma, particularly scaphoid fracture. Missed scaphoid fracture with displacement may result in avascular necrosis of the proximal portion of the scaphoid, due to its retrograde vascularization via the neck of the scaphoid. Clinically, there is usually restriction of flexion and extension of the joint with varying degrees of bony swelling, crepitus, and possibly synovitis. Radiographically, the features are the same as seen elsewhere, although there may be so-called scapholunate dissociation presumably as a result of damage to the interosseous ligaments by synovitis (**4.39**). Although unusual, other synovial joints in the hand and wrist may be affected.

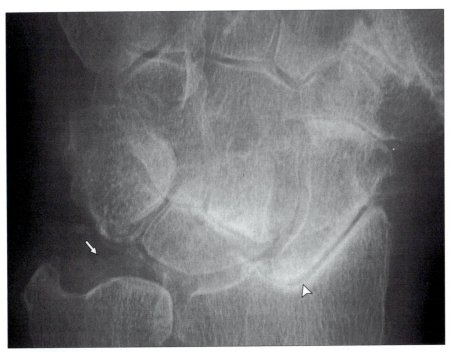

4.39 Wrist radiograph in pyrophosphate arthropathy showing chondrocalcinosis of the triangular ligament (arrow) and osteoarthritis of the radiocarpal, midcarpal, and scaphotrapezioid joints. Note the V-shaped depression in the distal radius (arrowhead) (associated with scapho-lunate dissociation) and marked bone attrition also in the proximal carpal row.

Features of osteoarthritis of the spine

Osteoarthritis of spine is often neglected in many studies of osteoarthritis. All the spinal synovial joints can be affected although some are targeted more than others. The most frequently affected are the apophyseal or facet joints, particularly in the lower cervical and lumbar spine. The clinical features of osteoarthritis of the facet joints can be difficult to correlate with the structural and radiographic abnormalities. Pain from spinal structures is often diffuse and hard to localize. Asymptomatic radiographic change is common and so attribution of symptoms to structural change is problematic. Indeed, provocation studies suggest that the pattern of pain produced by different spinal structures (joints, ligaments, discs, and muscles) can be similar if not identical. Previously, it was taught that pain on spinal extension was typical of lumbar facet joint osteoarthritis, but recent studies suggest that this is not the case, and there is no specific pain syndrome associated with facet joint arthritis.

Osteophyte formation can, however, be associated with encroachment of the neural foramina and subsequent impingement of the nerve root (4.40). This may produce a specific radiculopathy which may be provoked or aggravated by posture. Encroachment of the central canal may result in cord compression or symptoms of spinal claudication. This may be associated with ligamentum flavum hypertrophy and osteophyte formation at the site of the intervertebral disc insertion. This is discussed below when considering spondylosis.

Radiographically, facet joint arthropathy may be difficult to appreciate. On anteroposterior radiographs, sclerosis may be seen around the facet joints, and the presence of osteophyte may result in an apparent narrowing of the interpedicular distance as one looks caudally. On the lateral view sclerosis may be apparent, but the multiple overlapping bones and joints may make this difficult to evaluate. Foraminal encroachment may be observed, particularly if

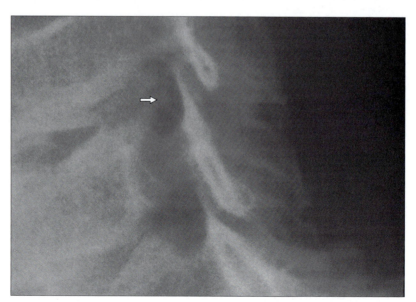

4.40 Foraminal encroachment resulting in nerve root compression in a patient with osteoarthritis of the cervical spine (arrow). Note difference in foraminal diameter between the involved superior foramen and the uninvolved lower foramen.

Features of osteoarthritis at specific sites

oblique views are taken centred on the foramen in question. There is no doubt that cross-sectional imaging, such as CT scanning and MRI scanning, is clearly superior in terms of evaluating structural change in osteoarthritis (4.41, 4.42). Although MRI scanning may detect oedema of the adjacent bone which may correlate with symptoms, these techniques essentially evaluate structure. Radioisotope scanning may detect increased bone turnover which, in turn, may correlate better with symptoms and response to local injection.

Other synovial joints in the spine, such as the atlantoaxial

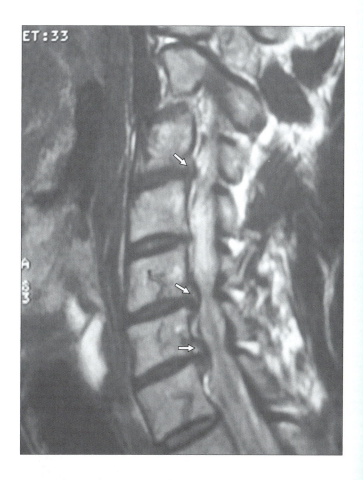

4.41 Lateral MRI scan of the neck. Loss of disc height and hydration is easily appreciated as blackening of the disc as well as posterior bony encroachment on the spinal cord (arrows).

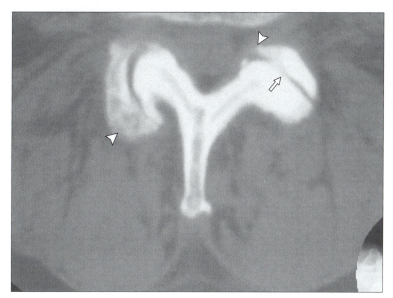

4.42 CT scan showing narrowing (arrow) and exuberant osteophytosis (arrowheads) of apophyseal joints.

76 Features of osteoarthritis at specific sites

joint and the atlanto-occiptal joints, may demonstrate features of osteoarthritis, but these are rarely clinically symptomatic. The joints of Lushka are the evolutionary remnants of the costotransverse joints of the cervical spine. The clinical consequences of involvement of these joints can be hard to determine, but osteophyte formation may cause impingement symptoms, such as dysphagia.

Occasionally, failure of segmentation of the spine may lead to additional joints, and these may develop features of osteoarthritis. A good example of this is the joint that may sometimes develop between the ilium of the pelvis and the transverse process of a lumbar vertebra.

While not a synovial joint, the discovertebral joint of the spine can develop features that have some similarities with osteoarthritis. Loss of hydration of the gelatinous nucleosus pulposus of the disc may result in loss of intervertebral height (**4.43**). Osteophytes may develop at the insertions of the annulus fibrosus and the longitudinal ligaments. These may simply produce a radiographic appearance which may be florid although often asymptomatic (**4.44**). It is likely that some disc changes, particularly if associated with bone marrow oedema, may cause pain. Large osteophytes may cause impingement on other structures. Anteriorly this may include the oesophagus, laterally the exiting nerve roots, and

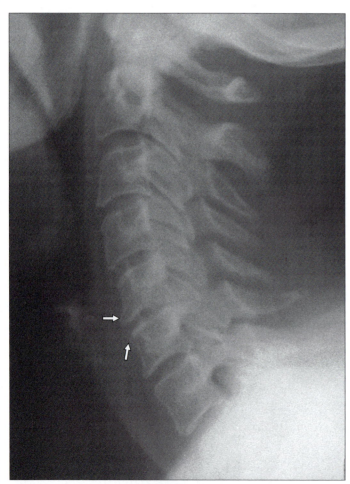

4.43 Lateral cervical spine radiograph showing intervertebral narrowing between the 5th and 6th cervical vertebra, with sclerosis and remodelling of the affected vertebrae (arrows).

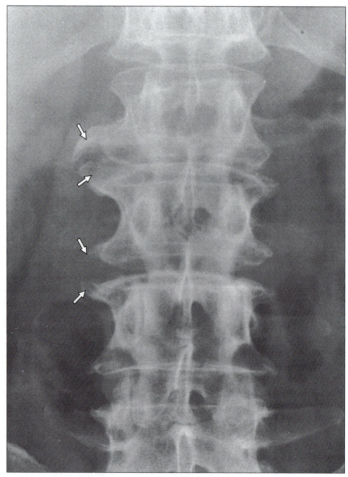

4.44 Lumbar spine radiograph showing narrowing at L2/L3 and L3/L4 and associated large lateral osteophytes arising from the vertebral end plates (arrows).

posteriorly it may encroach on the central canal. The shortening that results from loss of disc height may produce buckling of the longitudinal ligaments which further narrow the bony canal. Although frank cord compression may be produced with typical long-tract signs (in the lumbar region particularly), the syndrome of spinal claudication may also result.

Changes in the disc are often associated with facet joint arthropathy at the same level and this complex is often termed 'spondylosis', although this is a somewhat imprecise term and may be used differently by different clinicians. The issue as to whether facet joint osteoarthritis or disc degeneration is the initiating event is difficult, but most studies suggest that usually disc degeneration/dehydration occurs first. It is possible that the relative instability produced by the lost disc height increases stress on the facet joint and produces secondary osteoarthritic changes. Indeed, anteroposterior slippage may occur resulting in a spondylolisthesis (**4.45**).

Occasionally, there is loss of bone and a marked degenerative scoliosis may develop (**4.46**). Although this may cause major deformity, it may be surprising asymptomatic.

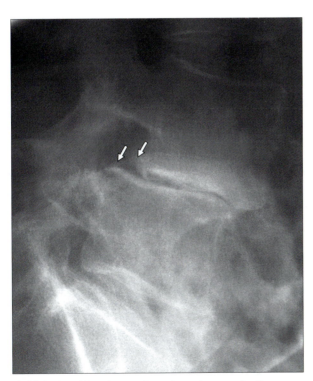

4.45 Lateral lumbar spine view demonstrating loss of disc height and a subsequent degenerative spondylolisthesis (arrows).

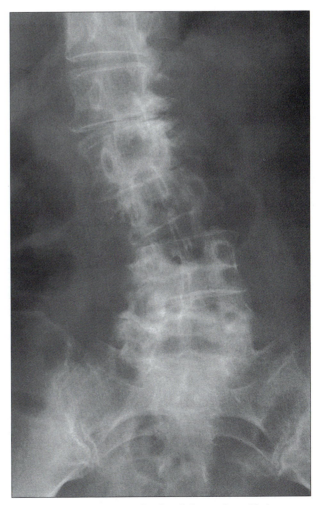

4.46 Degenerative scoliosis of the spine. Note the wedging of the lateral vertebral body and associated disc degeneration.

78 Features of osteoarthritis at specific sites

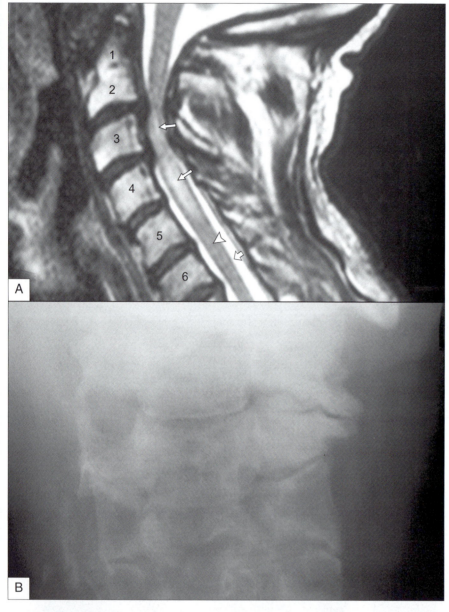

4.47 MRI scan of the cervical spine (**A**) showing osteophytosis disc degeneration and subsequent cord compression of the cervical cord at C2/3 and C3/4 (vertebral bodies are numberered). Indentation of the cord is clearly visible with loss of the surrounding high signal from the cerebrospinal fluid (normal anatomy shown: spinal cord [arrow head]; cerebrospinal fluid [short arrow]). In addition, there is high signal within the cord suggestive of cord oedema and/or ischaemia (arrows). The plain anteroposterior radiograph (**B**) demonstrates florid facet joint osteophytosis, narrowing, and sclerosis.

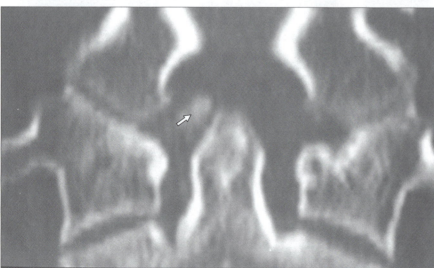

4.48 CT scan showing calcification due around the odontoid peg ('crowned dens syndrome') (arrow).

Spinal claudication is a clinical syndrome when exertion and/or spinal extension results in neurogenic pain, usually in the buttocks and perineum, and in more severe cases neurological dysfunction (**4.47**). On resting, this shows reversibility in the same way that claudication due to peripheral vascular disease does, though the time-scale for recovery is usually longer: 30 minutes compared to a few minutes. Clinically, it can be provoked by exercising the patient and evaluating neurological signs and symptoms before and after exercise. An alternative, and possibly simpler approach, is to hold the patient in lumbar extension for 2 minutes.

CPPD deposition can occur in the fibrocartilaginous discs and spinal ligaments. Occasionally, it occurs around the dens (**4.48**). Acute pseudogout episodes in relation to these deposits can cause self-limiting episodes of meningism, fever, neck and head ache, and sometimes confusion.

No discussion of osteoarthritis of the spine would be complete without a discussion of diffuse idiopathic skeletal hyperostosis (DISH or Forestier's disease). In this condition, there is flowing anterolateral paraspinal new bone formation that can bridge vertebrae and superficially resemble osteophytes or the syndesmophytes of ankylosing spondylitis. It particularly affects the right side of the thoracic spine (**4.49**) and both sides of the lumbar spine. In contrast to osteophyte, the underlying disc is usually structurally normal and the bridging new bone initially projects vertically rather than horizontally. It differs from syndesmophyte in that the new bone is almost layered onto the vertebrae (**4.50**), rather than arising from the annulus fibre insertions.

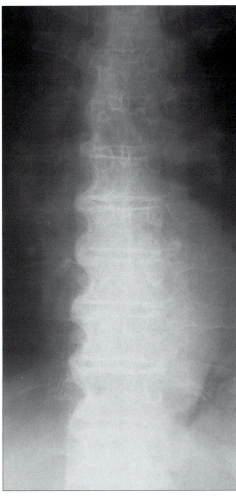

4.49 DISH. Flowing new bone formation bridging between vertebrae on the right side of the thoracic spine.

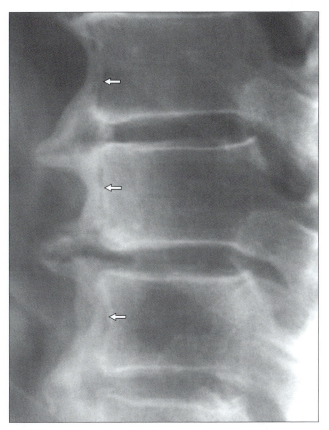

4.50 DISH. Lateral radiograph showing anterior new bone separate and 'layered' onto the anterior vertebral bodies. Note the initial projection of the osteophyte is away from the vertebral body rather than parallel to the annulus as is seen in ankylosing spondylitis. Note also 'cleft' between vertebral body and new bone (arrows). The intervertebral disc spaces are normal.

This diffuse hyperostosis may also occur at peripheral enthesis sites, particularly around the pelvis, knee, heel, and elbow (**4.51**). Symptoms that have been attributed to DISH included spinal stiffness and peripheral entheseal pain. The mechanism of the hyperostosis is unclear though DISH only occurs in middle-aged and elderly subjects and shows a strong association with obesity and type II diabetes.

The sacroiliac joint is part fibrous and part synovial. Although not a commonly appreciated problem, osteoarthritis of the sacroiliac joint does occur and may be difficult to distinguish radiographically from sacroiliitis seen in ankylosing spondylitis and the seronegative arthropathies.

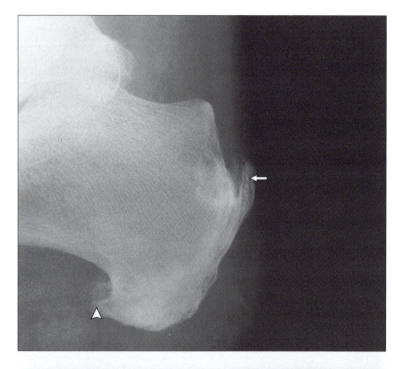

4.51 DISH. Lateral radiograph of the hindfoot showing exuberant new bone 'layered' over the back of the calcaneum and growing into the Achilles tendon (arrow) and plantar fascia insertion (arrowhead) sites. This patient had symptoms at both enthesis sites.

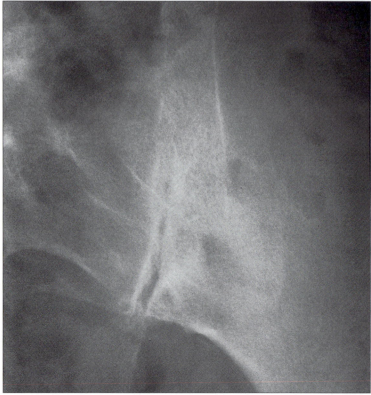

4.52 Radiograph showing osteoarthritis of the lower synovial part of the sacroiliac joint, with focal narrowing, sclerosis, and minor inferior osteophyte.

Features of osteoarthritis at specific sites

Irregularity of joint space width with sclerosis and inferior osteophyte are the typical x-ray features (**4.52**), and the early joint space widening, cortical erosion, and late ankylosis seen with sacroiliitis do not occur (**4.53**). Whether osteoarthritis of the sacroiliac joint is a common cause of symptoms is unclear.

Similar changes to that seen in the discovertebral joints may be seen in the symphysis pubis, another non-synovial, fibrous articulation. Sclerosis and apparent osteophyte formation are commonly seen, but it is unclear how much this is a normal developmental variation and how much a reaction to stress.

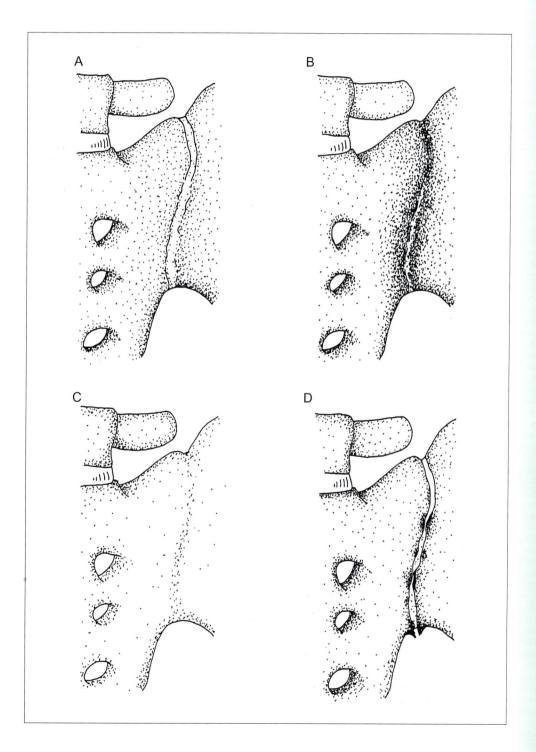

4.53 The first three diagrams are of sacroliliitis showing: (**A**) erosion of the cortical lines and initial apparent widening of the joint space; (**B**) progressive sclerosis and narrowing of the joint, still with ill-defined cortical lines; and (**C**) eventual obliteration of joint space and bony ankylosis. In contrast, the final diagram (**D**) shows osteoarthritis with focal narrowing, sclerosis, and inferior osteophyte with distinct cortical lines.

Features of osteoarthritis of the shoulder girdle

The shoulder girdle comprises the glenohumeral, acromioclavicular, and sternoclavicular joints, all of which may be affected by osteoarthritis.

Acromioclavicular joint osteoarthritis is a common cause of pain. This is localized over the joint and noted particularly on abduction of the shoulder. On examination, a superior arc of pain may be observed (**4.54**), and the simplest way to provoke the pain is with a scarf test – the shoulder is flexed to 90 degrees, and the arm adducted and internally rotated so the hand moves towards the opposite shoulder – with pain being felt principally over the apex of the shoulder. Crepitus can be felt on palpation during movement. Osteophyte can form superiorly where it can be palpated and may form a visible prominence (**4.55**). Chondrocalcinosis is another occasional cause of palpable swelling (**4.56**). Inferior osteophyte may impinge on the subacromial space and cause pain on abduction or stress of the supraspinatus muscle. Osteophyte formation and bony sclerosis may be difficult to appreciate on routine shoulder radiographs (which are usually designed to image the glenohumeral joint), but may be more apparent when dedicated acromioclavicular views are obtained. Associated degeneration of the underlying supraspinatus tendon may lead to rupture of the tendon and subsequent weakness of shoulder abduction.

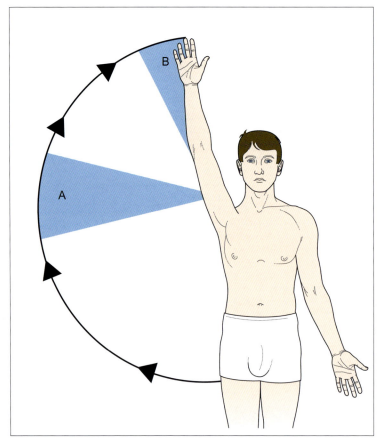

4.54 Two classic painful arcs. A painful middle arc (A) causes pain in the upper arm and may occur with either a supraspinatus lesion or subacromial bursitis. A painful superior arc (B) causes pain at the acromioclavicular joint site.

4.55 Prominent acromioclavicular joint swelling due to superior osteophyte.

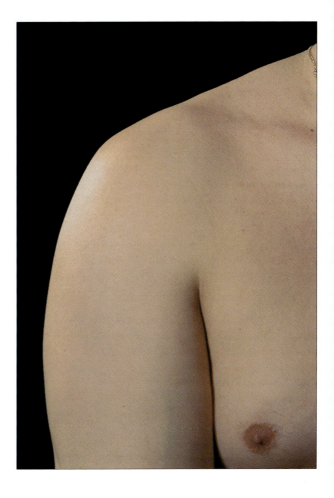

4.56 Exuberant chondrocalcinosis forming a palpable CPPD 'tophus' over the acromioclavicular joint (arrow).

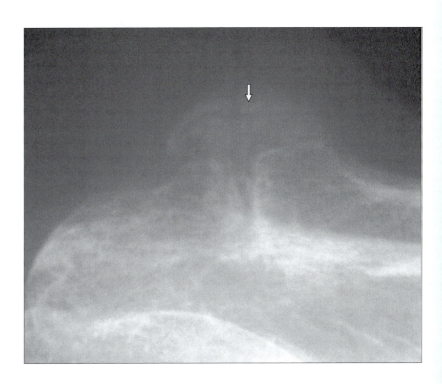

Features of osteoarthritis at specific sites

The glenohumeral joint is not a typical target site for osteoarthritis, but this may occur in the elderly, particularly in association with pyrophosphate arthropathy. This joint is also a target site for AADA or 'Milwaukee shoulder'. Glenohumeral pain is felt mainly in the dorsal aspect of the upper arm ('sergeant's stripes region', C5 dermatome), often occurring throughout the whole range of movement of the shoulder. There may be restriction of movement, especially abduction and external rotation and global muscle wasting. In addition, there may be associated rotator cuff disease with pain and possible weakness on resisted active movement (abduction – supraspinatus; external rotation – infraspinatus, teres minor; internal rotation – subscapularis (**4.57**). Acute crystal synovitis, due to CPPD (glenohumeral pseudogout) or apatite (acute calcific periarthritis), may lead to large glenohumeral and subacromial effusions, which may rupture and cause extensive bruising that tracks down the arm (**4.58**).

Radiographically, osteophytes may be appreciated most commonly on the inferior border of the glenoid, but also around the humeral head (**4.59**). However, joint space and subsequent flattening of the humeral head with sclerosis is often more readily appreciated, with an occasional additional finding of osteochondral bodies. Chondrocalcinosis of the hyaline cartilage and glenoid labrum may be seen radiographically, and apatite deposition in the superior rotator cuff ('calcific periarthritis') may also occur (**4.60**). If there is marked rotator cuff disease, the humeral head often migrates upwards (**4.61**).

Although the sternoclavicular joint commonly develops osteoarthritis, this is rarely a clinical problem. Ligamentous degeneration may result in subluxation of the joint and a bony prominence (**4.62**).

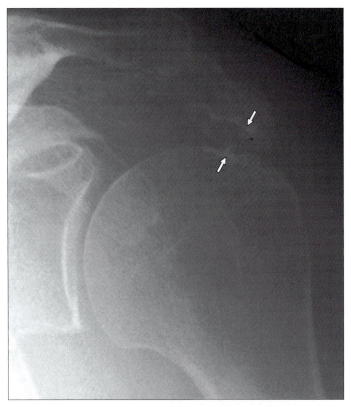

4.57 Anteroposterior radiograph of the shoulder. Note sclerosis (arrows) and encroachment laterally on the subacromial space which may result in symptoms of impingement on abduction.

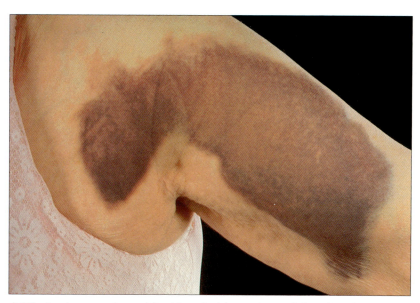

4.58 Acute pseudogout that has led to rupture of the glenohumeral capsule and subsequent bleeding and bruising down the arm. This can also occur with calcific arthritis.

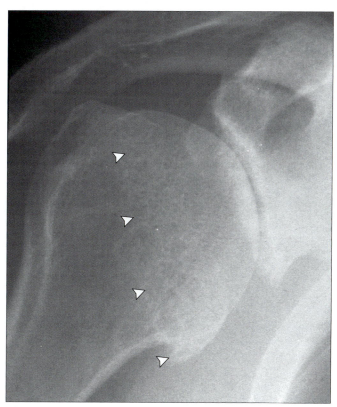

4.59 Glenohumeral osteoarthritis, showing narrowing, sclerosis, and a cuff of osteophyte around the margins of the humeral head (arrowheads).

86 Features of osteoarthritis at specific sites

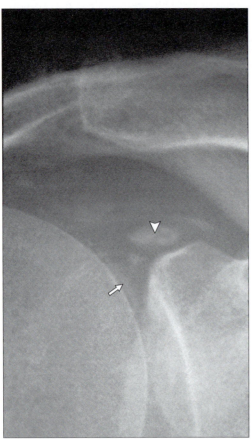

4.60 Chondrocalcinosis of hyaline cartilage forming a thin line close to, and parallel to the cortex of the humeral head (arrow). In addition, there is more dense deposits of apatite in the fibrous superior rotator cuff (arrowhead).

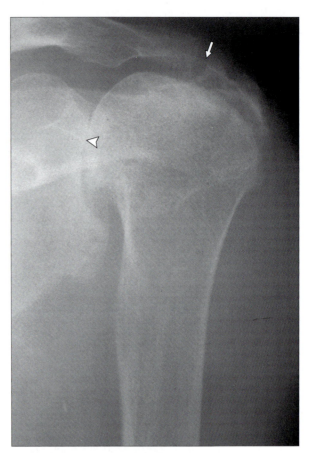

4.61 Glenohumeral osteoarthritis with associated rotator cuff degeneration and some associated widening of the acromioclavicular joint (arrow). Note joint space loss of the glenohumeral joint (arrowhead).

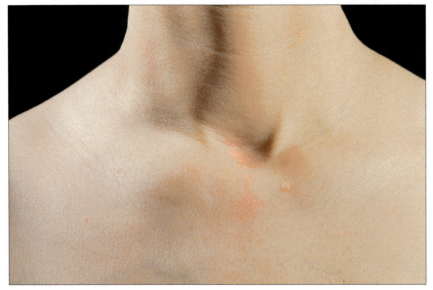

4.62 An asymptomatic sternoclavicular joint swelling due to osteoarthritis. Examination revealed bony swelling and crepitus on shrugging the right shoulder.

Features of osteoarthritis of the foot and ankle

Any joint of the foot and ankle may be affected, but again there is a predilection for certain joints.

Probably the most common joint affected is the 1st metatarsophalangeal joint of the hallux or big toe (**4.63**). This may occur as an isolated feature, but often is associated with so-called bunion formation (**4.64**). The principle features of a bunion are a marked valgus deformity of the proximal phalanx and formation of an adventitial bursa over the medial aspect of the joint. The major aetiological factor in bunion formation is probably varus alignment of the first metatarsal bone, usually as an inherited variation (**4.65**).

Clinically, there is pain over the joint, particularly on dorsiflexion of the hallux. Since dorsiflexion is necessary in the toe-off phase of gait, painful or poor mobility often results. On examination, there is restricted dorsiflexion, crepitus on movement, stress pain on dorsiflexing the toe,

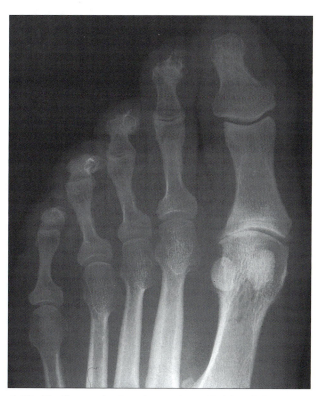

4.63 Radiograph showing osteoarthritis of the 1st metatarsophalangeal joint with focal narrowing, sclerosis and mild hallux valguus deformity.

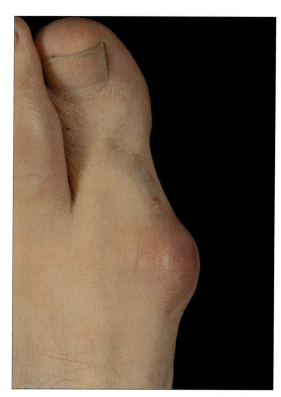

4.64 Bunion formation in a patient with hallux valgus due to osteoarthritis of the first metatarsophlangeal joint.

88 Features of osteoarthritis at specific sites

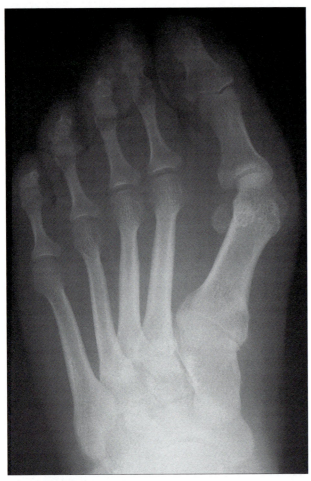

4.65 Radiograph showing metatarsus primus varus.

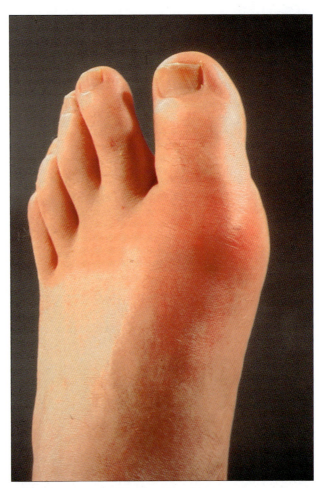

4.66 Acute gout affecting the 1st metatarsophalangeal joint – 'podagra'.

and bony swelling. If a bunion is present, the valgus alignment of the toe will be seen, and varying degrees of cystic bursal swelling or bony osteophytosis may be palpable. Occasionally, the bursa can become markedly inflamed with local heat and erythema. Gout has a predilection for damaged joints and a superimposed gouty arthritis may be developing (**4.66**).

The ankle mortise joint (between the tibia, fibula, and talus) may develop osteoarthritis, especially in the context of pyrophosphate arthropathy, and repetitive impact loading (parachuting) or trauma may be an overt aetiological factor. Pain in and around the ankle, particularly felt anteriorly, occurs on dorsiflexion. Involvement of the lateral or medial malleoli may result in pain on lateral or medial stress. Restriction of movement, particularly dorsiflexion, occurs in later disease and there may be varus or valgus hindfoot deformity. Radiographically, joint space narrowing can be appreciated; notably on anteroposterior views (**4.67**), although the loss of cartilage can be extremely focal. Osteophytes are more readily appreciated on the lateral view (**4.68**), and tend to occur on the anterior margin of the tibia and sometimes the talus. Other osteophytes may develop inferior to the medial and lateral malleoli.

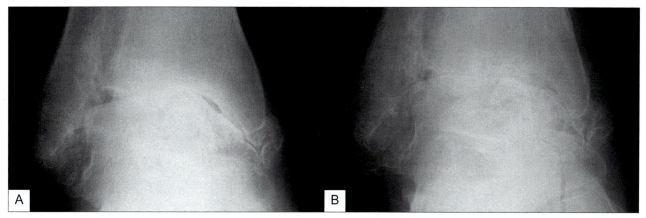

4.67 Anteroposterior views of right ankle joint of a man in his 60s with pyrophosphate arthopathy. The two views were taken just 3 years apart. Note the marked narrowing, sclerosis, deformity and osteophyte, and progressive bone attrition over this relatively short time.

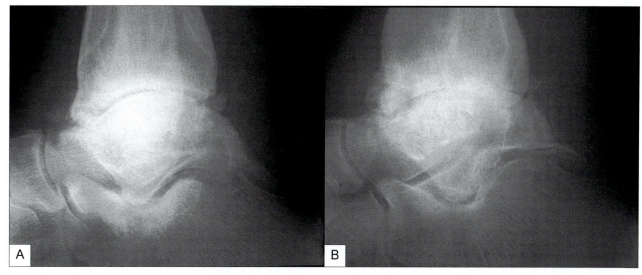

4.68 Lateral views of same patient as in **4.67**, again showing marked bone attrition over the 3-year period.

90 Features of osteoarthritis at specific sites

Subtalar involvement may be hard to establish, but can result in reduced eversion and inversion of the hindfoot with pain, especially when walking on uneven surfaces (**4.69**). Radiographically, sclerosis may be seen and occasional osteophytosis (**4.70**), although the complex shape of the joint can make assessment difficult.

Midtarsal joint involvement is not uncommon, especially in the context of pyrophosphate arthropathy. Although pronation and supination of the forefoot can be reduced, the major clinical feature is often osteophytes that develop over

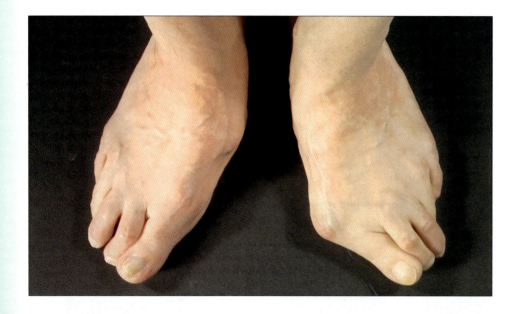

4.69 A 70-year-old man with subtalar and midfoot osteoarthritis and pyrophosphate arthritis of both knees. Note the eversion of both hindfeet, midfoot bony prominence and flat-footedness. He also has 1st metatarsophalangeal osteoarthritis and a marked left hallux valgus.

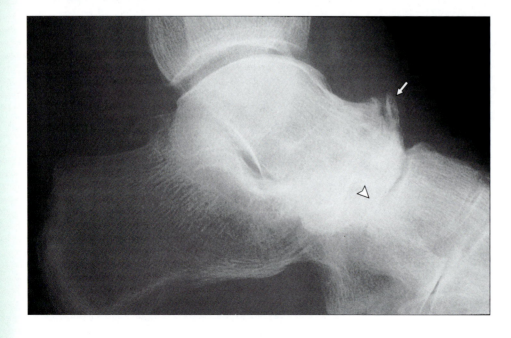

4.70 Radiograph showing subtalar osteoarthritis with narrowing, sclerosis (arrowhead), and superior osteophyte (arrow).

Features of osteoarthritis at specific sites

the dorsal aspect of the foot (**4.71, 4.72**). This can make fitting of footwear problematic and may lead to impingement of overlying tendons with pain on walking and movement of the toes. Radiographically, the osteophytosis can be readily appreciated, especially on lateral views, as well as some joint space narrowing (**4.72**), although again due to the complex nature of the joint specialized views or cross-sectional imaging may be required for full assessment.

Although other joints may be affected, these are not often a clinical problem.

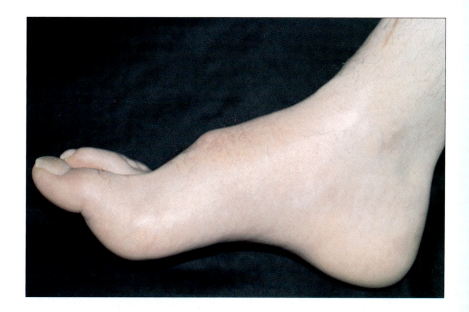

4.71 Midfoot osteophye causing prominent dorsal swelling.

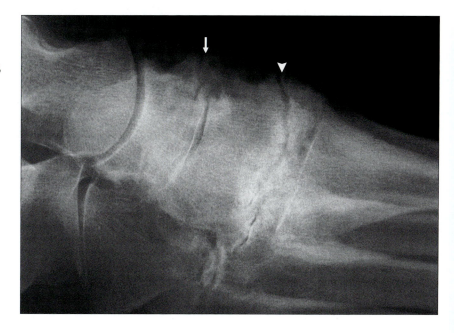

4.72 Radiograph showing osteoarthritis of the midtarsal (arrow) and tarsometatarsal joints (arrowhead) with narrowing, irregularity, sclerosis, and prominent dorsal osteophyte.

Features of osteoarthritis of the elbow

Osteoarthritis of the elbow is not commonly encountered, but this may be because it is often relatively asymptomatic. Trauma, including repetitive impact loading, may be a precipitating factor, especially in men, and an association with metacarpophalangeal osteoarthritis in men has been described. All three components of the joint (humeroulnar, humeroradial, and radioulnar) may be affected. Although pain may be a feature, for example, on extension or pronation/supination of the elbow, a relatively painless fixed flexion deformity is common. Crepitus may be seen, especially on palpation over the radioulnar joint during pronation/supination (4.73).

Radiographically, there is usually focal joint space narrowing and sclerosis (4.74, 4.75). Osteophyte is generally most apparent medially and laterally. Occasionally, anterior or posterior osteophyte may act as a physical block to extension, and flexion loose bodies may associate with locking.

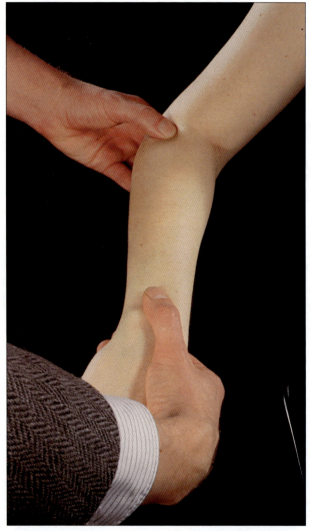

4.73 Palpation for crepitus over the proximal radioulnar joint during passive pronation/supination.

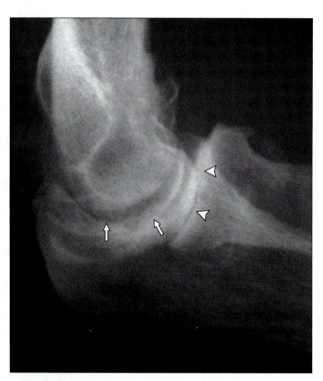

4.74 Lateral radiograph showing humeroulnar (arrows) and humeroradial osteoarthritis (arrowheads) with osteophyte, narrowing, sclerosis, and several anterior and posterior osteochondral bodies.

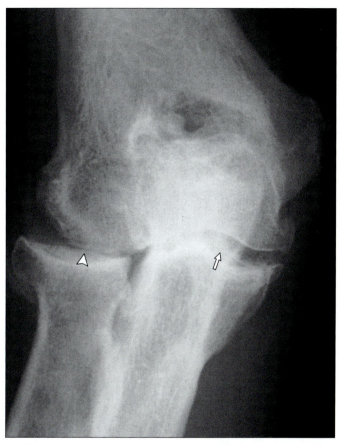

4.75 Anteroposterior view of elbow showing humeroulnar (arrow) and humeroradial (arrowhead) osteoarthritis with focal narrowing, sclerosis, and osteophyte.

Features of osteoarthritis of the jaw

The temporomandibular joint is a complex gliding joint, containing a fibrocartilaginous meniscus. Although commonly overlooked by rheumatologists, it is frequently affected by osteoarthritis. Associated meniscal degeneration is common.

Clinically there is pain, usually felt anterior to the ear, although it may radiate widely to the jaw, side of head, and even the neck and shoulder region. The range of movement may be affected with reduced mouth opening and lateral movement. Meniscal degeneration may result in locking, usually with the mouth open.

Dedicated imaging techniques are required to evaluate the joint and these may demonstrate joint space narrowing and sclerosis. Arthrography (and now more recently MRI scanning) may demonstrate meniscal degeneration and tears.

Further reading

Brandt KD, Doherty M, Lohmander LS (2003). *Osteoarthritis*, 2nd edn, Oxford University Press, Oxford.

Moskowitz RW, Howell DS, Altman RD, *et al.* (2001). *Osteoarthritis: Diagnosis and Medical/Surgical Management*. WB Saunders, London.

Resnich D, Niyama G (2002). *Diagnosis of the Bone Joint Disorders*, WB Saunders, London.

Chapter 5

Principles of management

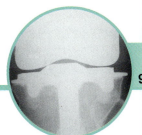

Introduction

In the management of osteoarthritis, there are several tools available (**5.1**). There are a wide number of options, including non-pharmacological, pharmacological, and surgical options, which may be selected and tried for the individual patient. The management plan has to be individualized, taking into account factors such as: severity of pain and disability; constitutional factors (e.g. obesity, muscle weakness); psychosocial factors; co-morbidity; concurrent drug therapy; and patient beliefs. With respect to choice of additional interventions, the evidence for efficacy is clearly important, although other factors that will guide decision-making include: the safety profile; the availability and practicality of the intervention; its mode of delivery; the cost of treatment; previous experience of the patient; and physician and patient preference.

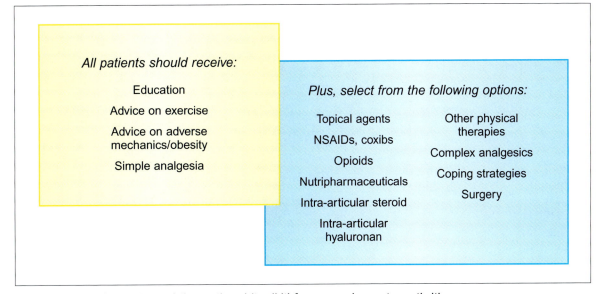

5.1 The core elements and the optional 'toolkit' for managing osteoarthritis.

Education

As with any chronic disease, patient education is paramount, particularly as evidence suggests that patients with high degrees of self-efficacy have better outcomes in terms of pain and disability. Ideally, education should take a cognitive approach, as enhanced problem-solving strategies and behaviours are the goal, rather than simple knowledge. A variety of approaches have been used, but essentially the fundamental principles are:

- Messages need to be given that are consistent.
- There needs to be an exploration of the patients beliefs and logical constructs so that the educational message is either not dissonant with this, or the underlying beliefs are challenged when required.
- Educational materials need to be culturally relevant and appropriate to the educational level of the recipient.

While these principles are easy to elucidate, putting them into practice is a considerable challenge within most health and social care services. Doctors and allied health-care professionals clearly have a role in this, but patients may receive a lot of their information and, indeed, possible misinformation from a number of sources (**5.2, 5.3**). There are a wide variety of sources that provide information on osteoarthritis (e.g. patient literature, interactive programmes, websites, and books). Many patients receive much of their education from non-professionals, such as friends and family. Education, therefore, may need to take place at a societal, as well as personal level. This is again a major public health challenge.

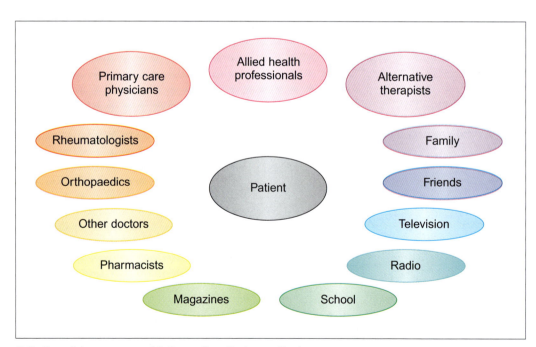

5.2 Possible sources of information that a patient may access.

Principles of management

5.3 Patient education and information access should be given to everyone with osteoarthritis.

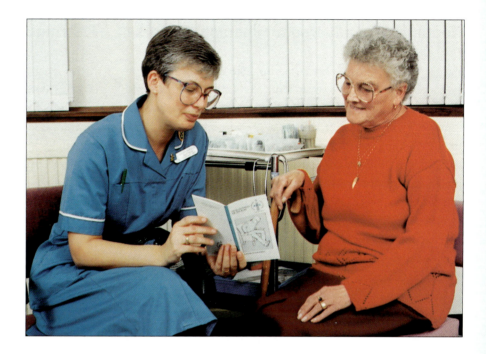

Exercise

Many recent studies have demonstrated that 'exercise therapies' can improve pain and disability in osteoarthritis, particularly that of the knee. There is still uncertainty as to the most appropriate exercise programme, but elements that emphasize aerobic fitness, proprioception, strengthening, and confidence all seem to be helpful. A major component may be the increase in self-belief and self-efficacy that follows, helping patients to view their osteoarthritis as a manageable process rather than a passive, degenerative, and inevitably progressive process (**5.4**).

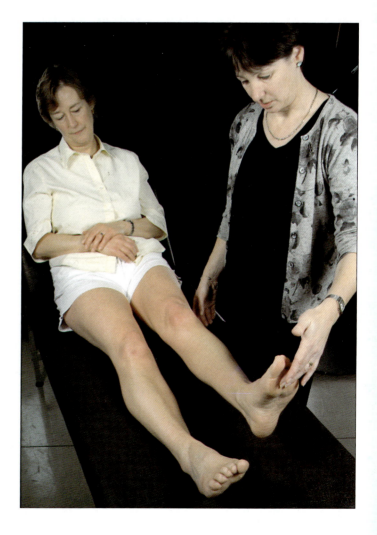

5.4 Patients should be encouraged to perform regular daily exercises to maintain movement and increase strength of the muscles that act over an osteoarthritic joint.

Reduction of adverse mechanical factors

Pacing of activities – breaking up activities into shorter episodes – can reduce strain on osteoarthritic joints, and allows tasks to be completed successfully. Appropriate footwear, with thick soft soles and no raised heels, reduces impact-loading on the feet, knees, hip, and spine (5.5). Adaptation of footwear can also alter mild valgus/varus malalignment and correction of leg length discrepancy. If the patient is overweight or obese, weight loss can improve symptoms and reduce risk of progression of knee and hip osteoarthritis. A walking stick, used correctly, can successfully reduce loading across a compromised knee or hip, and there are a wide range of orthoses that similarly can reduce adverse stress and improve symptoms and function.

Many other therapies have been suggested to be helpful for osteoarthritis at some sites, including: acupuncture; transcutaneous nerve stimulation; balneotherapy; passive physiotherapy modalities; osteopathy; chiropraxy; manipulative therapies; magnet therapy; homeopathy; dietary supplements; and herbal remedies. Although each has its devotees, the evidence for these various approaches is often not very strong. Nevertheless, a large number of patients will try one or more of these therapies, and so it behooves professionals to enquire and advise regarding them.

Pharmacological therapy

Most pharmacological approaches to therapy in osteoarthritis take a symptomatic approach, and all current analgesics have been employed in management. Paracetamol (acetaminophen) is the cornerstone of most guidelines regarding initial management because of its efficacy, low cost, and excellent safety in recommended dosage. If this is insufficient, other agents, particularly the non-steroidal anti-inflammatory drugs (NSAIDs) are used. Other alternatives for more severe pain include opioids, such as codeine, dihydrocodeine (alone, or with paracetamol), nefopam, tramadol, and meptazanol. For all patients with osteoarthritis, the important consideration is balancing efficacy of symptom control against the potential toxicity of the agent employed.

Surgery

There is no doubt that surgery, particularly prosthetic joint arthroplasty, has transformed the management of severe osteoarthritis (5.6). Problems remain, however. Not all joint sites are amenable to arthroplasty and, in essence, the hip and knee are really the only joints that are commonly

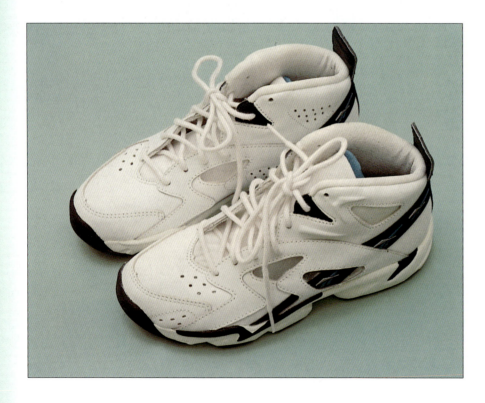

5.5 Many training shoes have the four qualities of a good shoe for arthritis: a thick, soft (air-filled) sole; no raised heel; broad forefoot; and soft, deep uppers. Increasingly, other fashion shoes with the same qualities are becoming available.

addressed by this approach. Even when a prosthesis is available, there are issues regarding the optimal design and method of fixation. The core of the problem is that long-term follow-up over many years is required before the true success of a prosthesis can be determined. No amount of *in vitro* testing can truly obviate the need for decades of clinical follow-up and assessment. The results can be critically confounded by surgical experience, perioperative management, and patient selection, and major questions remain as to the optimal approach.

Other surgical approaches are possible at some joint sites. For example, at the 1st metatarsophalangeal joint, non-prosthetic arthroplasty and excision arthroplasty is commonly used. At some painful joints, arthrodesis may be appropriate, and this is often employed at the thumb base, and even more so in the spine, where spinal fusion has long been used in an attempt to reduce pain.

Osteophytes can cause problems, in some circumstances, and examples of this include sub-acromial impingement in acromioclavicular osteoarthritis and neural compression, in and around the spine. Operations to decompress impingement and remove osteophyte can be successful in these circumstances.

Meniscal and ligamentous damage can be intimately associated with osteoarthritis. These clearly may need dealing with in their own right, with the added issue that interference with these structures may have an impact on the subsequent development of osteoarthritis. Minimally, invasive techniques have had a major impact on approaching these problems.

In recent years, the idea of 'joint repair' has gained ground. In essence this involves transplantation of tissues and tissue-engineering approaches in order to try to replace damaged tissues, especially cartilage. At present, the indications for this remain limited, and the process is still experimental.

Disease modification in osteoarthritis

The appreciation that osteoarthritis is a metabolically active process has lead to many attempts to develop strategies that promote the reparative aspects of the process and/or ameliorate the deleterious pathways. While a number of agents, some currently available for human use, have shown promise in this respect, it is probably fair to say that this approach still requires validation in humans.

Further reading

Brandt KD, Doherty M, Lohmander LS (2003). *Osteoarthritis*, 2nd edn, Oxford University Press, Oxford.

Felson DT (Conference Chair) (2000). Osteoarthritis: New Insights Part 1. The disease and its risk factors. *Ann Intern Med*, **133**:635–649.

Hosie DT, Dickson J (2000). *Managing Osteoarthritis in Primary Care*. Blackwell Science, Oxford.

Resnick D, Niyama G (2002). *Diagnosis of the Bone Joint Disorders*, WB Saunders, London.

Zhang W, Doherty M, Arden N, *et al.* EULAR evidence based recommendations for the management of hip oseoarthritis. *Ann Rheum Dis*, (in press).

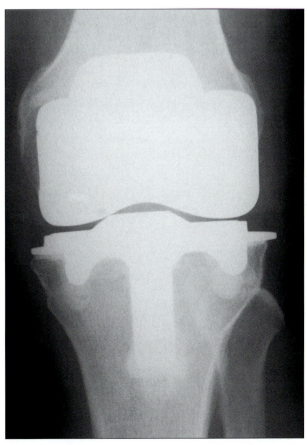

5.6 Joint arthroplasty at the knee with replacement of both the tibial and femoral joint components.

Appendices

Appendix 1: EULAR guidelines for the management of knee osteoarthritis

Final 10 key recommendations

- Use a combination of pharmacological and non-pharmacological measures.

- Tailor treatment according to symptoms, structural damage, location, and underlying risk factors.

- Use patient education, orthoses, and aim to reduce obesity.

- Use paracetamol (acetaminophen) as the mainstay of pain relief.

- Use topical agents (non-steroidal anti-inflammatory drugs (NSAIDs)/capsaicin).

- Use oral NSAIDs in unresponsive patients and select on the basis of safety: use COX 2 selective drugs 'coxibs' or co-prescription of gastroprotective agents where required.

- Use opiod analgesia if required or where NSAIDs are contra-indicated or not tolerated.

- Slow-acting osteoarthritis drugs, including glucosamine sulphate and hyaluronans, may aid symptoms and may be structure modifying.

- Intra-articular corticosteroids may have short-term benefits.

- Joint replacement surgery should be considered in patients with pain and disability in spite of the above measures.

Adapted from: Jordan KM, Arden NK, Doherty M, *et al.* (2003). EULAR Recommendations 2003: an evidence based approach to the management of knee osteoarthritis: Report of a Task Force of the Standing Committee for International Clinical Studies Including Therapeutic Trials (ESCISIT). *Ann Rheum Dis,* **62**: 1145–1155.

Appendix 2: American College of Rheumatology guidelines for the management of hip and knee osteoarthritis

- Non-pharmacological measures should include education, weight loss, exercise therapy, orthoses, social support, and advice on joint protection.

- Pharmacological therapies should include NSAIDs, paracetamol (acetaminophen), opioids, and topical agents.

- The choice of pharmacological agent should be individualized to the patient according to preference, severity of symptoms and the risk of toxicity.

- Gastroprotective agents and safer agents (coxibs) should be considered.

- Intra-articular hyaluronan injections should be considered, particularly if NSAIDs are contra-indicated.

- Intra-articular corticosteroids may be indicated for acute exacerbations of pain particularly if there is associated clinical evidence of inflammation.

- Opioid agents should be considered.

- Tidal irrigation of the knee joint may be effective in some patients but the results of larger trials are awaited.

- Surgery should be considered in patients who fail to respond to conservative measures.

Adapted from: Altman RD, Hochberg MC, *et al.* (2000). Recommendations for the medical management of osteoarthrits of the hip and knee. *Arth Rheum*, **43**: 1905–1915

Index

Note: page numbers in **bold** refer to illustrations and those in *italics* to tables or boxes

acetabular dysplasia 14, **15**, 66
acetaminophen (paracetamol) 98
acromegaly 17–18, **19**
acromioclavicular joint 82, **86**
age 6
American College of Rheumatology (ACR) 24, *102*
analgesics 98
animal models 4
animals, non-human 5
ankle joint 18, 88–91
ankylosis, bony 70, 81
ankylosis human (ANKH) gene 48
apatite associated destructive arthritis (AADA) 49, **50–1**, 59, **60**, 84
arthritis, primary inflammatory 14, 59, **60**
arthrography 93
arthroplasty 99
asymptomatic osteoarthritis 22
avascular necrosis (osteonecrosis) 18, **19**, 31, 64, 73

Baker's (popliteal) cyst 53
basic calcium phosphate (BCP) crystals 49
blood vessels **3**
body weight 7
bone loss **3**, 20, 31, 35, **37**
  in AADA 49, **51**
bone marrow oedema 38, 76
bone response 2
  see also osteophyte formation
Bouchard's nodes 42, 68
bruising 84, **85**
bunion formation 87
'buttressing' 35, **36**

calcific periarthritis 84
calcium pyrophosphate dihydrate (CPPD) deposition 20–1, *32*, 44–8
  ankle 88, **89**
  knee 59, **60**
  metabolic diseases predisposing to 46–7
  patterns of joint involvement *46*
  shoulder **83**, 84
  spine 79

cartilage loss 1, 20, **21**
  assessment and grading 26–7, **28**, 34, **35**
  see also joint space narrowing
childhood disorders 14
chondrocalcinosis 44–8
  familial 48
  hip 64, **65**
  knee **45**, 56, **59**
  metabolic diseases predisposing to 46–7
  shoulder 82, **83**, **86**
  wrist 73
co-morbidity 20
computed tomography (CT) 75, **78**
cortical buttressing 64
crepitus 26, 54, 82, 92
'crowned dens syndrome' **78**, 79
cyst, popliteal 53
cyst formation 17, **18**, 20, **21**, 35, **36**, **37**
  hip osteoarthritis 6, **63**, **65**
  knee 59
  wrist **18**, 72

'decompensated' osteoarthritis 29
definitions of osteoarthritis 1–3, 20, 24
deformity 26
  foot 87, **88**
  hip 61
  knee 54, 56, **58**
'degenerative disease' 29
diffuse idiopathic skeletal hyperostosis (DISH) 79, **80**
discovertebral joint 76
disease modification 5, 99
distal interphalangeal joints 6, 41–2, 67–8
diuretic therapy 68
dysplasia
  acetabular 14, **15**, 66
  epiphyseal/spondyloepiphyseal 16

education, patient 96, **97**
elbow 33, 92, **93**
endemic osteoarthritis 17
enthesophyte 56, **58**
epidemiology 4, 5–19, 20
erosive osteoarthritis 43, 70
European League Against Rheumatism (EULAR) guidelines 101
evolutionary perspectives 29

exercise therapies 97

facet joint osteoarthritis 74, 77
femoral condyle, medial 18, **19**
femoral head **2**, 18, **19**, **21**
fibrocartilage, intra-articular 22
fixed flexion deformity, knee 54
flexion deformity, hip 61
foot 80, 87–91
footwear 98
Forestier's disease 79

gender 6
generalized nodal osteoarthritis 4, 6, 9, 41–2
genetic factors 9–10, **11**, 46–8
'giving way' 33
glenohumeral joint 33, 84, **85**, **86**
gout 44, 68, **69**, 88
'gull's wing' sign 70

haemochromatosis 17, **18**, 35, 46–8, 64, **65**, 72, 73
hallux valgus 87, **90**
hand osteoarthritis 7, 12, 17, 67–73
Heberden, William 9
Heberden's nodes 9, 41–2, 67–8, **69**
hip dysplasia 14, **15**, 66
hip osteoarthritis **2**, 61–6
  AADA 51
  cyst formation 6, **63**, **65**
  factors in progression 66
  joint space narrowing 1, **37**, 62, **63**
  osteonecrosis 18, **19**
  osteophyte formation **2**, 35, **36**, 62, 64
  pain 61
  patterns of 62, **63**
  risk factors 6, 12, 15
history of osteoarthritis 4–5
'hook' osteophytes **72**, 73
hyperostosis, diffuse idiopathic skeletal (DISH) 79, **80**
hyperparathyroidism *47*
'hypertrophic' osteoarthritis **2**, 46
hypomagnesaemia *47*
hypophosphatasia *47*

imaging techniques 38–9
  jaw 93
  knee 56

imaging techniques (*continued*)
  spine 74–5, 79
information, patient 96

jaw osteoarthritis 93
joint capsule **3**
joint effusions
  glenohumeral joint 84, **85**
  knee 53
  shoulder 49, **50**
joint repair 99
joint space narrowing 1
  ankle joint 88, **89**
  elbow 92
  glenohumeral joint **86**
  grading 26–7, **28**
  hand and wrist 68, 71
  hip **1**, **37**, 62, **63**
  knee 55
  midfoot 91
  radiographic assessment 34, **35**, 37
  spine 76, **80–1**
joint swelling 32, 82, **83**, **86**
joint usage 12

Kashin–Beck disease 17
Kellgren and Lawrence grading system 26, 27
knee, joint replacement 99
knee osteoarthritis 2, **3**, **36**, **45**, 53–60
  ACR definition 24
  bone marrow oedema 38
  factors in progression 39
  imaging 39, 56
  pyrophosphate deposition **44–5**
  risk factors 6, 7, 8, **11**, 12, 13, 14

Lesquesne Algofunctional Index 26
ligaments 22
ligamentum flavum hypertrophy 74
'locking' 33–4, 56
loose bodies 33, **37**, 92
Lushka, joints of 76

magnetic resonance imaging (MRI) 38, 75, **78**, 93
management 95–7
  guidelines 101–2
  pharmacological 98
  surgical 99
mechanical factors, reduction of adverse 98
meniscal injury 8, 9, 22, **23**, 99
meniscectomy 22
menopause 6, 9, 67
metabolic disease 7, 17–19, 35, 46–8, 64, **65**, **72**, 73
metabolic syndrome 20
metacarpophalangeal joints 71, **72**
metatarsus primus varus 87, **88**
'micro-klutziness' 14
midfoot 90–1
midtarsal joint 90, **91**
'Milwaukee' shoulder 49, 84
'Missouri arthropathy' 71
Modic change 38
monosodium urate crystals **69**

mortality 20
muscle strength 13
muscle wastage 26, 33, 62

nail dystrophy 67
neurological risk factors 14
nodal generalized osteoarthritis 4, 6, 9, 41–2
nodes, *see* Bouchard's nodes; Heberden's nodes
non-steroidal anti-inflammatory drugs (NSAIDs) 98

obesity 7
occupation 12, 71
opioids 98, 101
osteochondral bodies 18, 33, **37**, 56, **58**, 64, 92
osteonecrosis 19, 31, 35, 64, 73
osteophyte formation 2, 20, **21**, 31
  ankle 88, **89**
  early, cartilaginous 35
  elbow 92, **93**
  hand and wrist **72**, 73
  hip **2**, 35, **36**, 62, 64
  imaging 35, 36
  knee **2**, **21**, 55, 56, **57**, **58**
  midfoot 90–1
  as repair process 29
  shoulder girdle 82, **83**, 84, **85**
  spine 74, 75, 76–7, **80–1**
  surgical management 99

Paget's disease 14, **15**, 66
pain 22–4, 31
  causes 25
  hand and wrist 70
  hip 61
  jaw 93
  nocturnal 31
  pharmacological management 98
  shoulder 82
  spinal osteoarthritis 74, 79
  variation in intensity 24, **25**
paracetamol (acetaminophen) 98
patellofemoral joint 2, **3**, **36**
Perthe's disease 14
pharmacological therapy 98
'podagra' 88
Pond–Nuki model 4
popliteal cyst 53
progression, factors in 38, 39, 46
protrusio acetabulae 62, **63**
pseudogout 32, 44, 47, 84, **85**
pyrophosphate arthropathy, *see* calcium pyrophosphate dihydrate (CPPD) deposition

quadriceps tendon, patella insertion 56, **58**

radiographic features 34–5, **36–7**
  assessment and grading 34–5, **36–7**
radioisotope scanning 39, 75
'regenerative joint disease' 5, 29
rheumatoid arthritis 14, 59, 60
risk factors 6–19, **11**
rotator cuff disease 84, **86**

sacroiliac joint 80, **81**
'saw-tooth' deformity **36**
scapholunate dissociation 73
scaphotrapezoid joint 71
sclerosis **2**, 35, **36**, 68, 80–1, 90, 92, **93**
scoliosis 61, 77
sex hormones 6
shoes 98
shoulder girdle 33, 49, **50**, 82–6
sibling studies 10, **11**
'skier's knees' 54
spinal claudication 77, 79
spinal cord compression 74, 77
spinal osteoarthritis 74–81
  diffuse idiopathic skeletal hyperostosis 79, 80
  sacroiliac joint 80, **81**
spondylolisthesis, degenerative 77
spondylosis, spinal 77
sport 12
sternoclavicular joint 84, **85**, 86
steroid therapy 18, **19**
stiffness 26, 32
stroke 14
subsets of osteoarthritis 40, 41
  erosive osteoarthritis 43, 70
  generalized nodal osteoarthritis 41–2
  pyrophosphate arthropathy 44–8
subtalar osteoarthritis 90
surgery 98–9
symphysis pubis 64, **65**, 81
symptoms 22–4, **25**
  assessment 24–6
synovitis 20–2, 53, 59

temporomandibular joint 93
tendons 22, 56, **58**
'thumb base' squaring 70
tissues, involved in osteoarthritis 2, **3**
tophi 68, **69**, 83
toxins 17–18, **19**
trapeziometacarpophalangeal joints 71
trauma 8, 9, 12
twin studies 10

ultrasound scanning 39

'vacuum' phenomenon 77
valgus deformity
  foot 87
  knee 54, 59, **60**
varus deformity
  first metatarsal 87, **88**
  knee 54, 56, 59

Western Ontario and McMasters Universities (WOMAC) Osteoarthritis Index 26
whales 5
'windswept' knees 54
wrist 17, **18**, 67–73

young onset osteoarthritis 9, 16, 18, *20*, 51